HEAD AND NECK RADIOLOGY

Arnold Noyek, MD, FRCS(C), FAC
Professor of Otolaryngology and Radiology
University of Toronto
Staff Otolaryngologist and Radiologist
Department of Otolaryngology
Mount Sinai Hospital and Sunnybrook Medical Centre
Toronto, Ontario, Canada

J. B. Lippincott Company • Philadelphia
Gower Medical Publishing • New York • London

Distributed in USA and Canada by:
J.B. Lippincott Company
East Washington Square
Philadelphia, PA 19105
USA

Distributed in the rest of the world (except Japan) by:
Gower Medical Publishing
Middlesex House
34-42 Cleveland Street
London W1P 5FB
UK

Distributed in Japan by:
Nankodo Company Ltd.
42-6, Hongo 3-Chome
Bunkyo-Ku
Tokyo 113
Japan

10 9 8 7 6 5 4 3 2 1

Library of Congress Cataloging-in-Publication Data
Noyek, Arnold M.
    Head and neck radiology / Arnold Noyek.
        p.   cm.
    Includes bibliographical references and index.
    ISBN 1–56375–002–3
    1. Head—Radiography.   2. Neck—Radiography.
I. Title.
    [DNLM: 1. Head—radiography.   2. Neck—
radiography.. WE 705 N937h]
RC936.N68   1991
617.5'10757—dc20
DNLM/DLC
for Library of Congress   91-10560
                          CIP

British Library Cataloguing in Publication Data
Noyek, Arnold
    Head and neck radiology
    1. Humans. Head. Radiology.
    I. Title
    616.0757
    ISBN 1–56375–002–3

Editors: Bill Gabello, Patrick D. O'Neill
Art Director: Jill Feltham
Illustrator: Alan Landau, Seward Hung
Designer: Nava Anav

Printed in Hong Kong
Produced by Mandarin Offset

CONTENTS

INTRODUCTION   **V**

CHAPTER ONE
Temporal Bone   **1**

CHAPTER TWO
Paranasal Sinuses   **15**

CHAPTER THREE
The Nasopharynx   **35**

CHAPTER FOUR
Orbital Extension of Diseases
of the Nasal Cavity and
Paranasal Sinuses   **39**

CHAPTER FIVE
Skull Base   **43**

CHAPTER SIX
Intracranial Relationships of
Otorhinologic Disorders   **47**

CHAPTER SEVEN
Maxillofacial Skeleton   **51**

CHAPTER EIGHT
Temporomandibular Joints and
Mandible   **57**

CHAPTER NINE
Major Salivary Glands   **63**

CHAPTER TEN
Thyroid Gland   **71**

CHAPTER ELEVEN
Parathyroid Glands   **77**

CHAPTER TWELVE
Superior Mediastinum   **79**

CHAPTER THIRTEEN
The Larynx and Cervical Trachea   **83**

CHAPTER FOURTEEN
Upper Digestive Tract   **91**

CHAPTER FIFTEEN
Vascular Lesions of the Head
and Neck   **97**

CHAPTER SIXTEEN
Nonvascular Soft-tissue Lesions
of the Neck   **101**

CHAPTER SEVENTEEN
Otolaryngologic Manifestations
of Systemic Disease   **107**

BIBLIOGRAPHY   **B.1**

INDEX   **I.1**

INTRODUCTION

Diagnostic imaging provides a unique perspective of the patient, his disease, its complications, and its response to treatment. This is particularly true in the field of otolaryngology–head and neck surgery, which deals with the most complex anatomic region in the body. Much head and neck disease lies within visceral spaces or bony structures, and is inaccessible to direct inspection even with state-of-the-art telescopes or endoscopes.

The newer high-tech imaging modalities have had a major impact on head and neck diagnosis. Computed tomography (CT) has revolutionized the management of malignant disease. In patients with advanced (T3 and T4) malignancies, it is now possible to document the extent of the primary disease. (The same concept applies to any patient with a tumor of the head and neck that cannot be fully and accurately staged by clinical means.) The presence—or absence—of lymph node metastases can be ascertained with a high degree of confidence. Armed with this information, the clinician can make a realistic choice among various treatment options. Follow-up CT scans enable the clinician to assess the results of treatment and compare the efficacy of various treatment methods.

The advent of high-resolution sonography has had a major impact on thyroid diagnosis. Technical refinements in nuclear medicine have increased our understanding of the biologic aspects of many disease processes. Magnetic resonance imaging (MRI)—the newest and perhaps the most exciting diagnostic tool in our armamentarium—promises to have a major impact in many areas of soft-tissue imaging, though its precise role remains to be defined. Despite these technical advances, conventional bread-and-butter radiology continues to play a central role in head and neck diagnosis.

An imaging work-up should be carefully tailored to the clinical problem. The choice of imaging studies, and the sequence in which they are done, should be the joint decision of the referring physician and a radiologist with special expertise and interest in one or more aspects of head and neck imaging. Cost-effectiveness and risk–benefit ratio have become important considerations. Some patients require no studies at all; others require simple conventional radiographic examinations; and still others require an extensive investigation, which may entail costly high-tech examinations, as well as invasive procedures (e.g., angiography, sialography) that carry an inherent risk. A poorly performed study—whether due to technical deficiencies or inadequate active monitoring—may be worse than no study at all. Inadequate studies can lead to misdiagnosis or mismanagement; there should be no hesitancy to repeat them. In the context of other diagnostic studies, a carefully planned and executed imaging work-up will enable the clinician to formulate a reasonable working diagnosis and answer several fundamental questions.

1. What is the qualitative diagnosis? This may be a specific diagnostic label (e.g., fracture, osteoma) or a more general diagnostic category (e.g., bone-destructive, cystic, or vascular disease).
2. What is the quantitative diagnosis? Does the disease extend beyond specific anatomic boundaries (e.g., orbital extension of a paranasal sinus infection)? What are the precise relations of the fragments in a complex maxillofacial fracture?
3. Do any specific findings suggest a specific pathologic diagnosis? A hot thyroid nodule is likely to be a functioning adenoma; a hot parotid mass is probably a Warthin's tumor; a highly vascular neck mass is most likely a paraganglioma, hemangioma, or arteriovascular malformation.
4. What is the physiologic status of the disease? For example, if osteomyelitis is present, is it active or quiescent?
5. Is there a specific structural abnormality (e.g., cerebrospinal fluid leak, arteriovenous malformation)? Can it be accurately localized?

In the chapters that follow, imaging techniques appropriate to various anatomic regions and clinical problems will be illustrated. It should be emphasized that head and neck imaging is a rapidly evolving field and a number of concepts presented here are in flux. As our understanding of the strengths and weaknesses of the newer imaging techniques increases, and as new technology comes along, many diagnostic pathways in vogue today will surely be modified.

Temporal Bone

The temporal bone houses the most complex anatomy in the body, with many important anatomic structures lying within millimeters of one another (Fig. 1.1). The middle-ear cleft, with its ossicles and air-cell system, overlies the cochlear and labyrinthine end organs in the rock-hard petrosa. The internal carotid artery (via the carotid canal) and the jugular foramen share important vascular relations with the temporal bone. Lesser vessels such as the ascending pharyngeal artery, which supplies the highly vascular glomus tympanicum and glomus jugulare tumors, and the occipital artery, which often supplies arteriovenous malformations, are intimately related to the temporal bone. Eight cranial nerves (5 through 12) pass through foramina or canaliculi in or adjacent to the temporal bone. Acoustic neuromas commonly arise from the vestibular segment of the 8th nerve, beginning as "ear" tumors within the internal auditory canal. The facial nerve has an extremely complex course through the temporal bone and may be affected by trauma, osteomyelitis, or tumor.

Cerebellopontine angle lesions are intimately related to the porus acousticus. Meningiomas and subarachnoid cysts typically arise in the vicinity of the porus. Acoustic neuromas arising within the internal auditory canal usually grow outward to reach the level of the porus and may extend intracranially to become "brain" tumors. The temporal bone is affected by a great variety of lesions arising in the middle or posterior cranial fossa.

Imaging of the temporal bone dates back to the first half of the twentieth century when Schuller, Owen, Law, Stenver, and Towne, among others, devised radiographic projections that projected the temporal bone away from other bony structures. By identifying bone destruction in the key attic/aditus/antrum region of the middle-ear cleft and lysis in the septate cellular structure of the mastoid, it became possible to diagnose inflammatory disorders that required surgical intervention (e.g., acute coalescent mastoiditis, cholesteatoma, tuberculous mastoiditis). Similarly, the late erosive changes associated with large acoustic neuromas could be identified radiographically (Fig. 1.2).

Before the advent of complex-motion thin-section tomography (polytomography) in the 1960s, pneumoencephalography and positive contrast cisternography—sometimes painful and hazardous procedures—were needed to demonstrate small acoustic neuromas. Complex-motion tomography represented a major advance in temporal bone imaging. Not only could bone destruction be detected at an earlier stage (Figs. 1.3, 1.4), but fracture relations could be seen more clearly

(Fig. 1.5); traumatic disruption of the ossicular chain, otosclerosis, and many congenital malformations (Fig. 1.6) became "radiologic" diagnoses for the first time.

The impact of CT on temporal bone diagnosis has been profound. Destructive lesions, as well as intracranial extension of inflammatory and neoplastic processes, are clearly depicted on unenhanced scans (Fig. 1.7); contrast enhancement may provide important additional information (Fig. 1.8). By using air or metrizamide as an intrathecal contrast agent, small tumors of the cerebellopontine angle and posterior fossa can be demonstrated (Fig. 1.9). With the sophisticated software now available on third and fourth generation scanners, it is now possible to obtain ultrathin (1 mm) cuts that depict normal anatomy and pathology more clearly than complex-motion tomograms and offer the added dimension of soft-tissue imaging (Figs. 1.10, 1.11). MRI

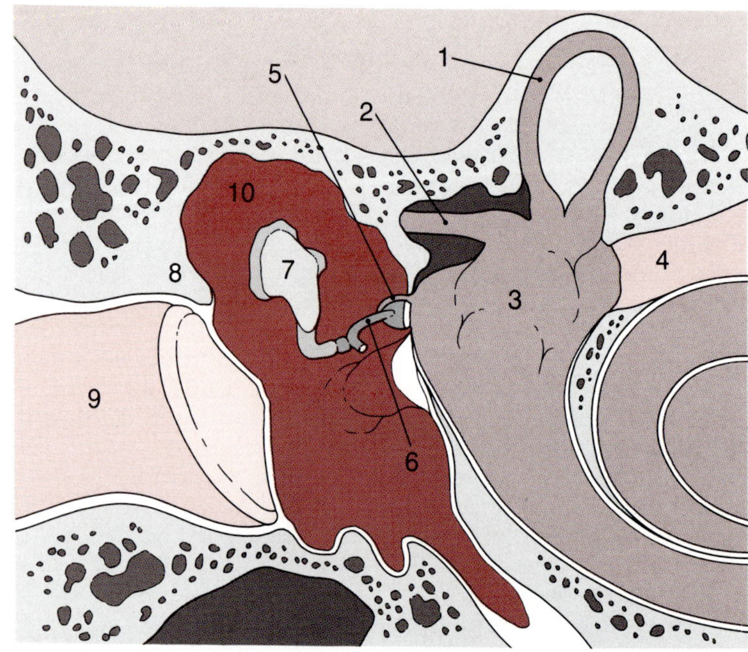

1 Superior semicircular canal	13 7th cranial nerve
2 Horizontal semicircular canal	14 Branches of 8th cranial nerve
3 Vestibule	15 Greater superficial petrosal nerve
4 Internal auditory canal	16 Geniculate ganglion
5 Foramen ovale	17 Labyrinthine segment, 7th cranical nerve
6 Stapes superstructure	18 Horizontal segment, 7th cranial nerve
7 Incus body and long process	19 Posterior semicircular canal
8 Scutum	20 Vestibular aqueduct
9 External auditory canal	21 Jugular foramen
10 Epitympanic recess	22 Foramen magnum
11 Internal carotid artery	
12 Cochlea	

promises to provide even more exquisite soft-tissue detail, allowing earlier diagnosis of acoustic neuroma and lesions of the facial nerve (Fig. 1.12).

Superselective angiography, augmented by digital subtraction techniques where appropriate, allows detailed study of the vascular anatomy of the temporal bone and posterior fossa. Intra-arterial embolization has been employed as a primary treatment modality or as a surgical "assist" in a growing number of patients with vascular lesions and tumors (Fig. 1.13).

Radionuclide bone scans and gallium scans are useful in the diagnosis and management of patients with osteomyelitis of the temporal bone and malignant external otitis (osteomyelitis of the external auditory canal). By obtaining serial studies, the "biologic stage" of the bone infection, as well as the response to treatment, can be assessed (Fig. 1.14).

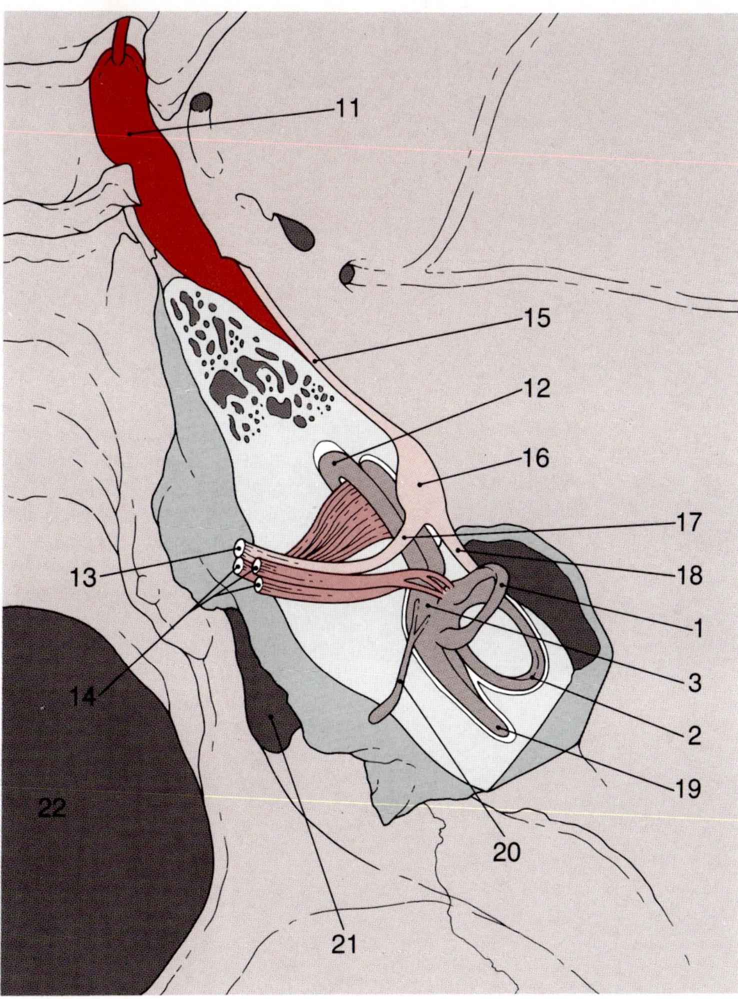

Fig. 1.1 Anatomy of the temporal bone. a *Schematic drawing showing the normal anatomy of the middle and inner ear at the level of the oval window. (Modified from Mancuso, Hanafee, 1985.)* **b** *Neural structures of petrous portion of temporal bone, viewed from above (corresponds to axial projection of CT or MRI examination). The overlying bone has been removed to display the 7th and 8th nerves and the semicircular canals. (Modified from Daniels DL et al, 1984.)*

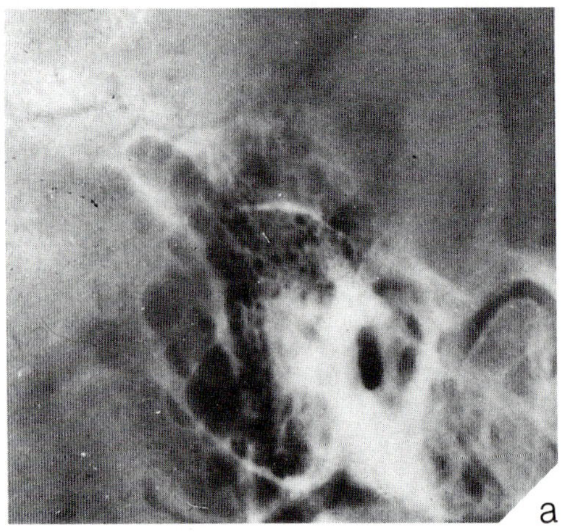
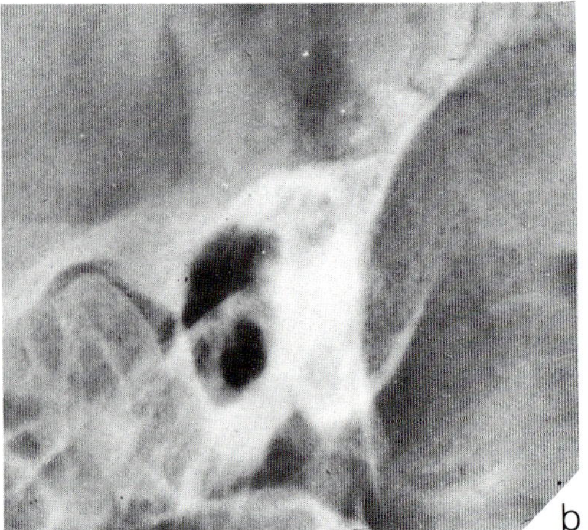
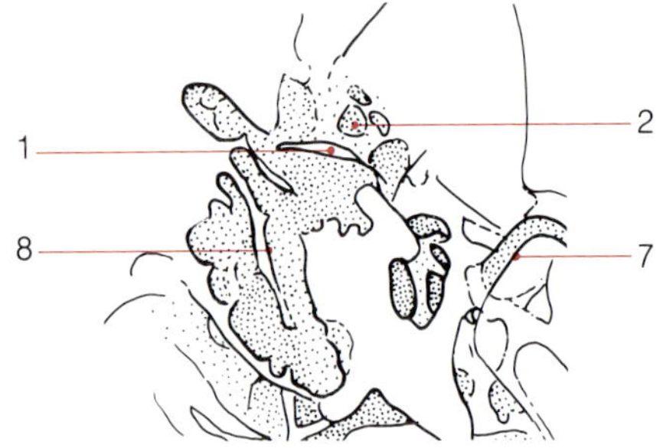
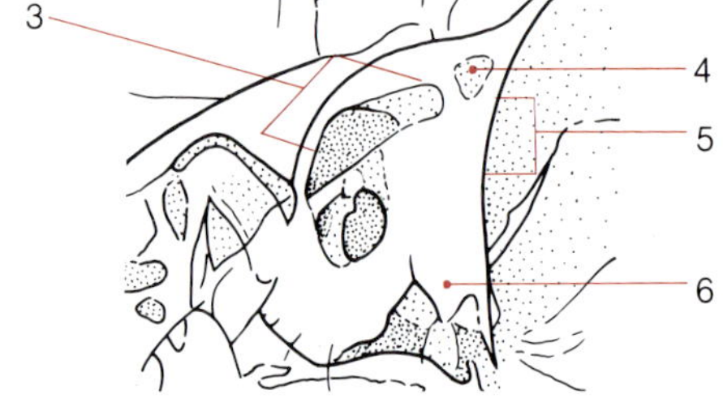

1	Tegmen plate	5	Sigmoid sinus plate
2	Normally pneumatized air cells in squamous portion of temporal bone	6	Sclerotic mastoid bone
3	Margins of cholesteatoma	7	Mandibular condyle
4	Opacified mastoid air cells	8	Sigmoid sinus plate

Fig. 1.2 Primary acquired cholesteatoma of the epitympanum (attic) and mastoid antrum. *a Schuller projection of normal side.* ***b*** *Schuller projection of diseased side shows a sclerotic mastoid bone (sharply outlined against the sigmoid sinus plate) with an expansile area of bone destruction representing a cholesteatoma. Opacified (obstructed) mastoid cells appear as a lucent focus adjacent to the cholesteatoma. (Note: The sclerotic appearance of the mastoid is due to underdevelopment of air cells resulting from inflammatory disease in early childhood, and does not indicate the presence of active infection.)*

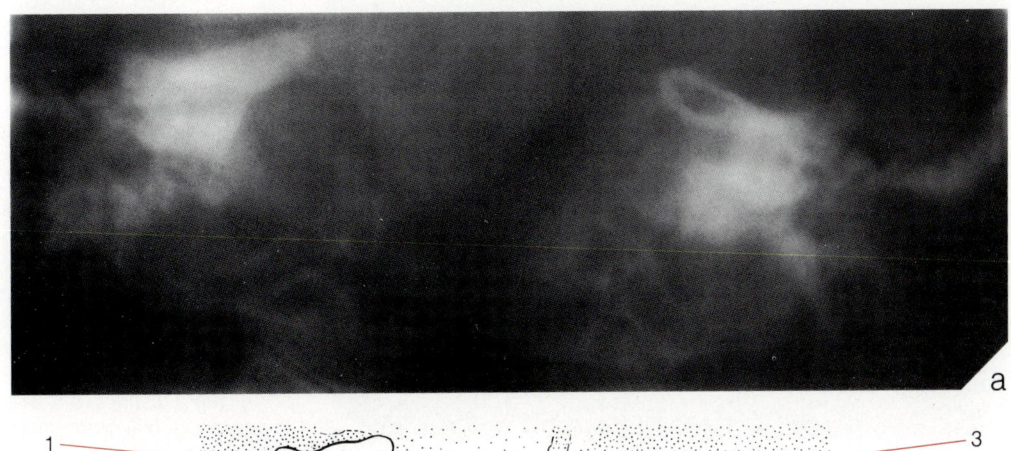

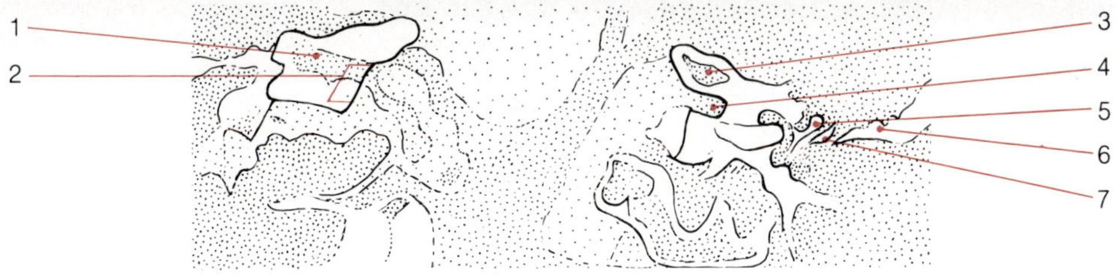

1 Internal auditory canal
2 Amputation of petrous apex
3 Petrous apex air cells
4 Internal auditory canal

5 Ossicle
6 Roof of external auditory canal
7 Tympanic spur
8 Destructive lesion

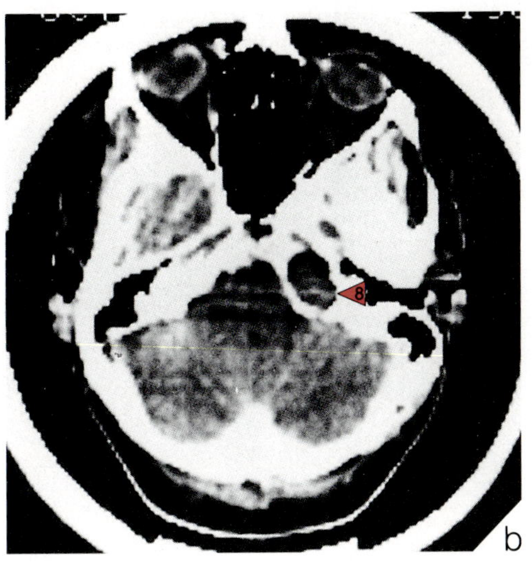

Fig. 1.3 Congenital cholesteatoma of the petrous apex. *a A complex-motion tomogram (coronal projection) shows normal morphology on the left. (On these and subsequent complex-motion tomograms the individual cuts are 1 mm thick.) On the right, the petrous apex is sharply amputated. The central portion of the right internal auditory canal has been destroyed as well. b The cystic nature of the destructive lesion (arrow 8) is apparent in this early-generation computed tomography (CT) scan.*

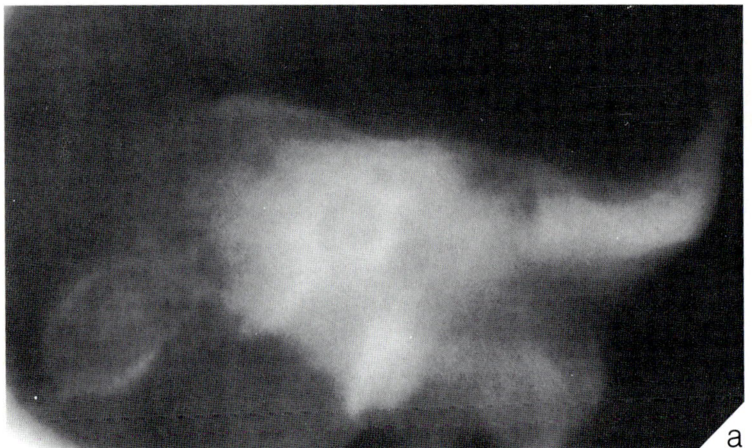

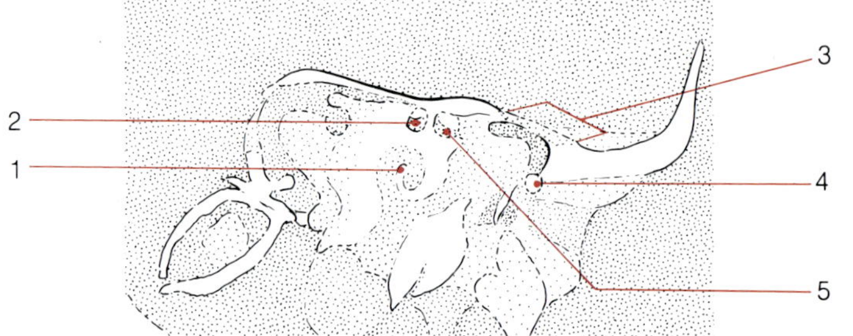

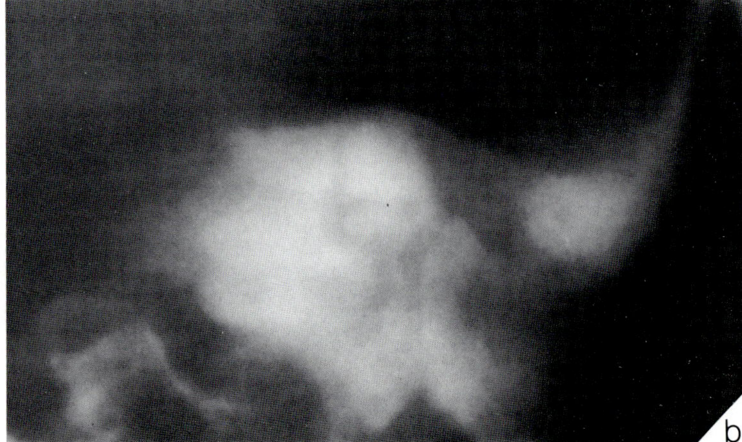

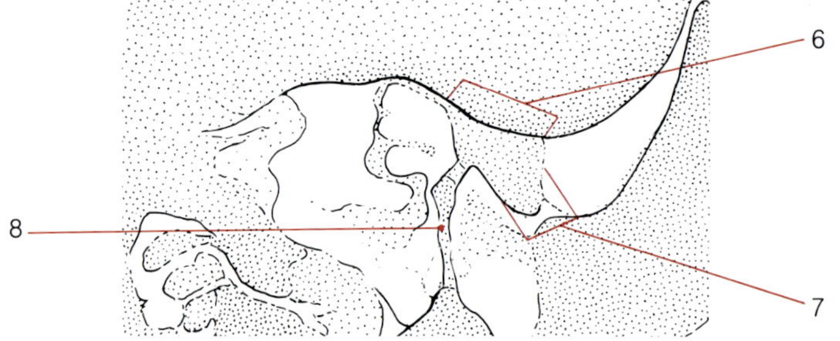

Fig. 1.4 Primary acquired cholesteatoma with extension Into the attic and mastoid antrum. *Complex-motion tomograms of the left petrous bone.* ***a*** *A coronal projection at the level of the cochlea demonstrates a large destructive focus (cholesteatoma) that extends superiorly into the attic. The bony tympanic spur has been destroyed. In this plane (close to the geniculate ganglion), the labyrinthine and tympanic segments of the bony facial nerve canal lie side-by-side, producing a distinctive "owl's eye" appearance.* ***b*** *A more posterior tomographic cut, at the level of the vestibule and superior semicircular canal, shows the superior extent, as well as the neck, of the cholesteatoma. The vertical segment of the bony facial nerve canal, which exits at the stylomastoid foramen, is also seen at this level.*

1 Cochlea
2 Labyrinthine segment of facial nerve
3 Margins of cholesteatoma
4 Tympanic spur
5 Tympanic segment of facial nerve
6 Cholesteatoma
7 Neck of cholesteatoma sac
8 Vertical segment of bony facial nerve canal

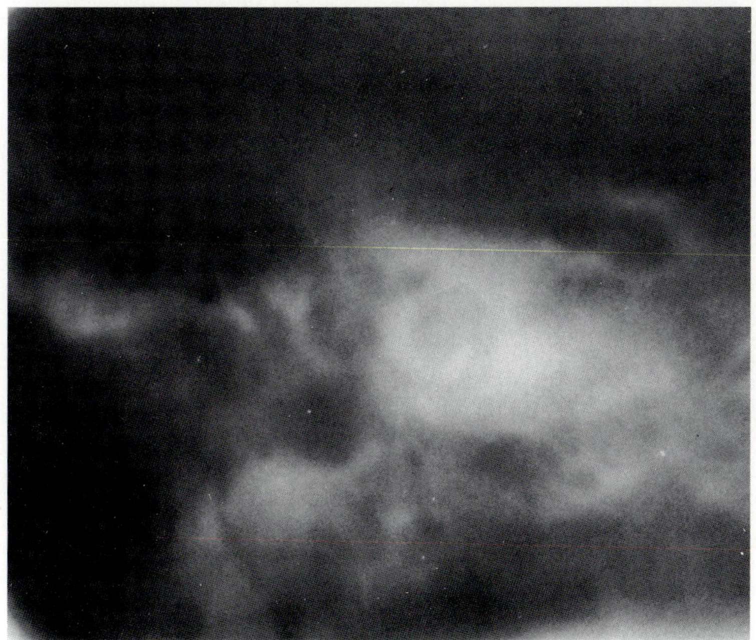

Fig. 1.5 Fracture of the floor of the external auditory canal.
Complex-motion tomogram of the right petrous bone. A coronal projection at the level of the cochlea demonstrates a fracture through the external auditory canal. The interval between the head of the malleus and the tympanic spur is increased in this longitudinal fracture. The middle-ear cleft is partially opacified by hemorrhage. (Reproduced with permission from Zizmor, Noyek, 1978).

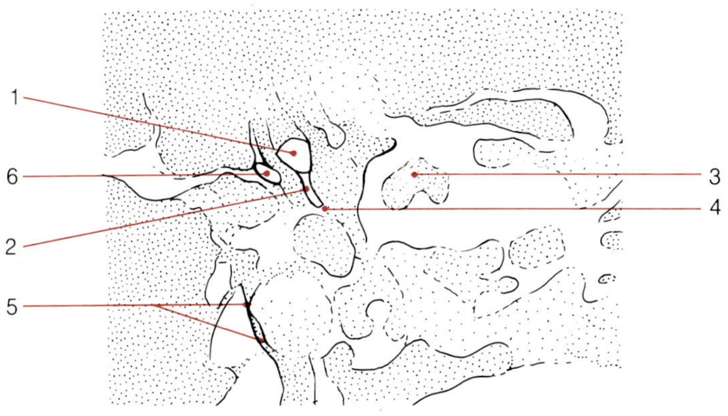

1	Malleus head	4	Blood in middle ear cleft
2	Malleus handle	5	Fracture
3	Cochlea	6	Tympanic spur

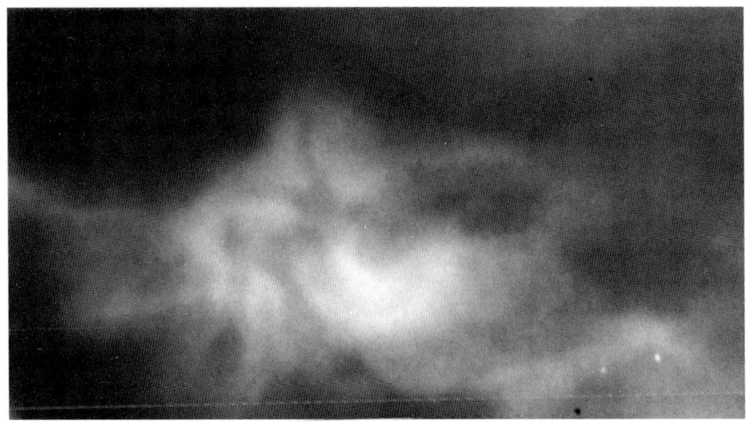

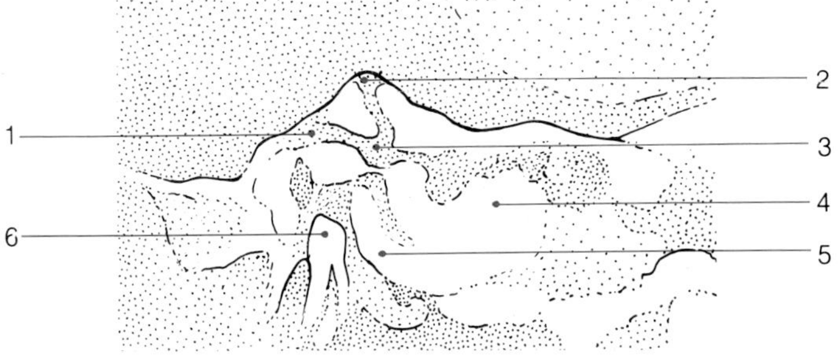

Fig. 1.6 Congenital bony atresia of the external auditory canal. *A complex-motion tomogram (coronal projection) of the right petrous bone in a patient with severe conductive hearing loss shows a bony plate obstructing the external auditory canal. In addition, there is bony mass within the middle-ear cavity. Other tomographic cuts (not shown) demonstrated deformity of the ossicular chain.*

1 Lateral semicircular canal
2 Superior semicircular canal
3 Vestibule
4 Basal turn of cochlea
5 Bony mass in middle ear cavity
6 Bony atresia

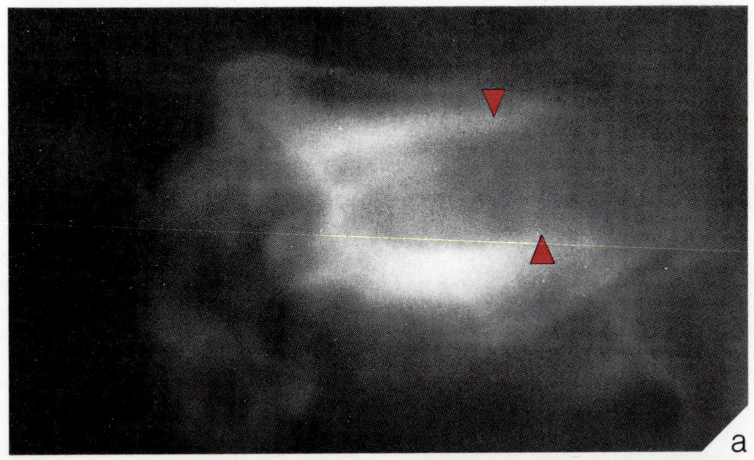

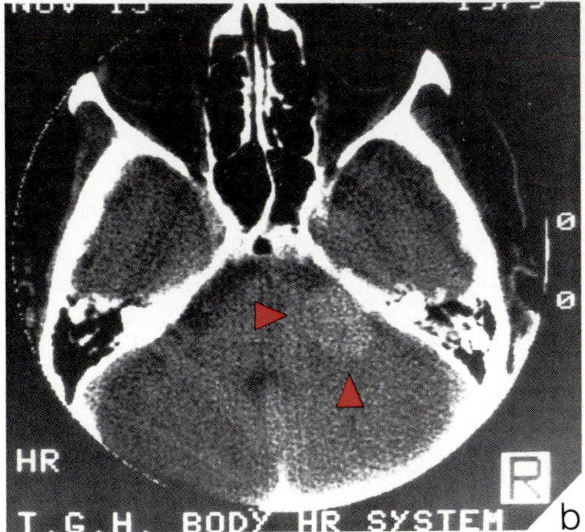

Fig. 1.7 Acoustic neuroma with bone destruction. *This 57-year-old woman presented with a progressive sensorineural hearing loss on the right side. **a** A complex-motion tomogram of the right petrous pyramid shows expansion of the porus acousticus (arrows). **b** An early-generation CT scan shows an enhancing mass (arrows) in the right cerebellopontine angle. The tumor originates within the internal auditory canal and projects into the posterior fossa. **c** Bone window of the cut in **b** shows erosion of the petrous pyramid (arrows) by the cerebellopontine angle tumor. (Note: As an acoustic neuroma grows it may or may not expand and erode the internal auditory canal. Because complex-motion tomograms may be normal even when the tumor has extended into the cerebellopontine angle, this technique is no longer acceptable for evaluation of sensorineural hearing loss.)*

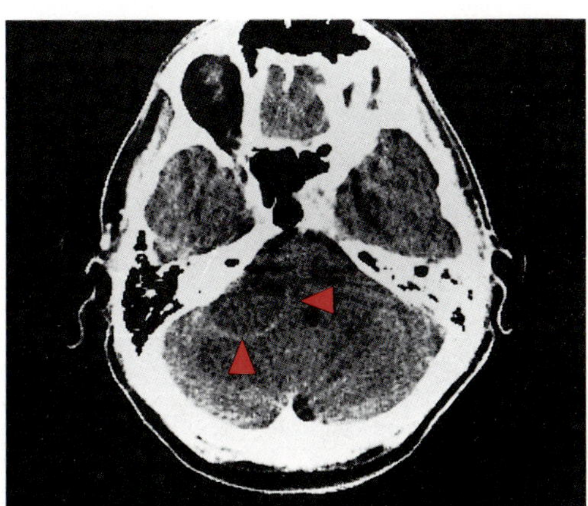

Fig. 1.8 Acoustic neuroma with enhancing rim. *This 48-year-old man presented with a progressive sensorineural hearing loss on the right. A contrast-enhanced CT scan shows a right cerebellopontine angle mass with an enhancing rim (arrows). The mass is of relatively low density, suggesting a cystic lesion; however at surgery it proved to be a solid acoustic neuroma. Rim enhancement reflects increased vascularity at the periphery of the lesion; it occurs in many inflammatory, neoplastic, and vascular lesions, and is of little help in differential diagnosis.*

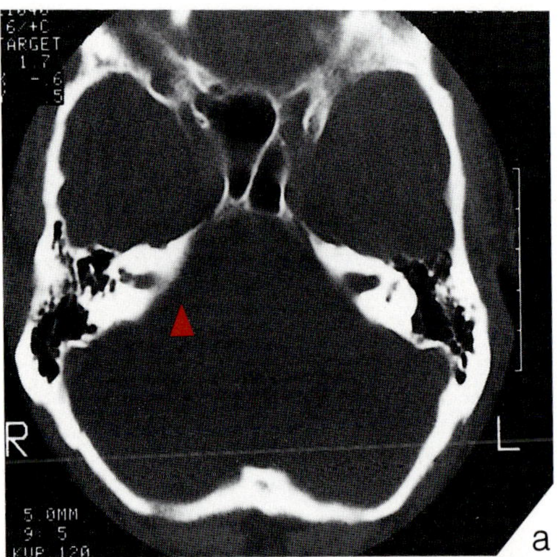

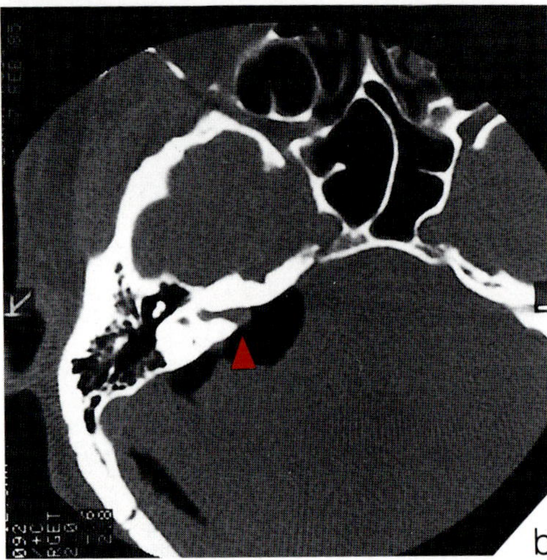

Fig. 1.9 Small acoustic neuroma. *a* Contrast-enhanced CT scan in a patient with a progressive right side sensorineural hearing loss, and an abnormal brainstem shows no abnormality at the cerebellopontine angle (arrow). *b* Repeat CT scan, with patient in left decubitus position, following intrathecal injection of air shows a soft-tissue mass (arrow) *within the internal auditory canal. The convex margin of the mass, which projects just beyond the porus acousticus, is exquisitely outlined by air. Very careful positioning of the patient is needed to maneuver air into the cerebellopontine angle to demonstrate tumors this small.*

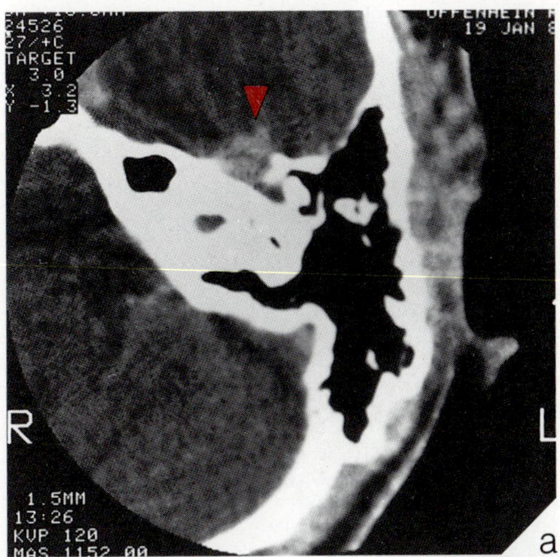

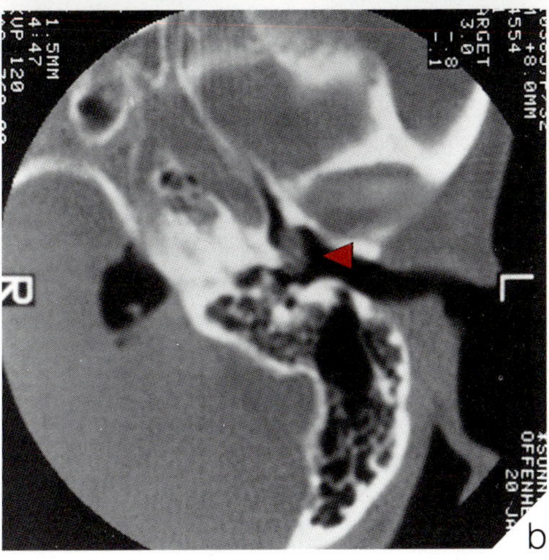

Fig. 1.10 Schwannoma of the facial nerve.
a High-resolution axial contrast-enhanced CT scan of the left petrous pyramid in a 29-year-old female with a partial peripheral facial nerve paralysis shows bone destruction in the region of the geniculate ganglion. An enhancing mass (arrow) projects into the middle cranial fossa.
b A more caudal cut demonstrates a soft-tissue mass (arrow), *outlined by air, within the middle-ear cleft.*

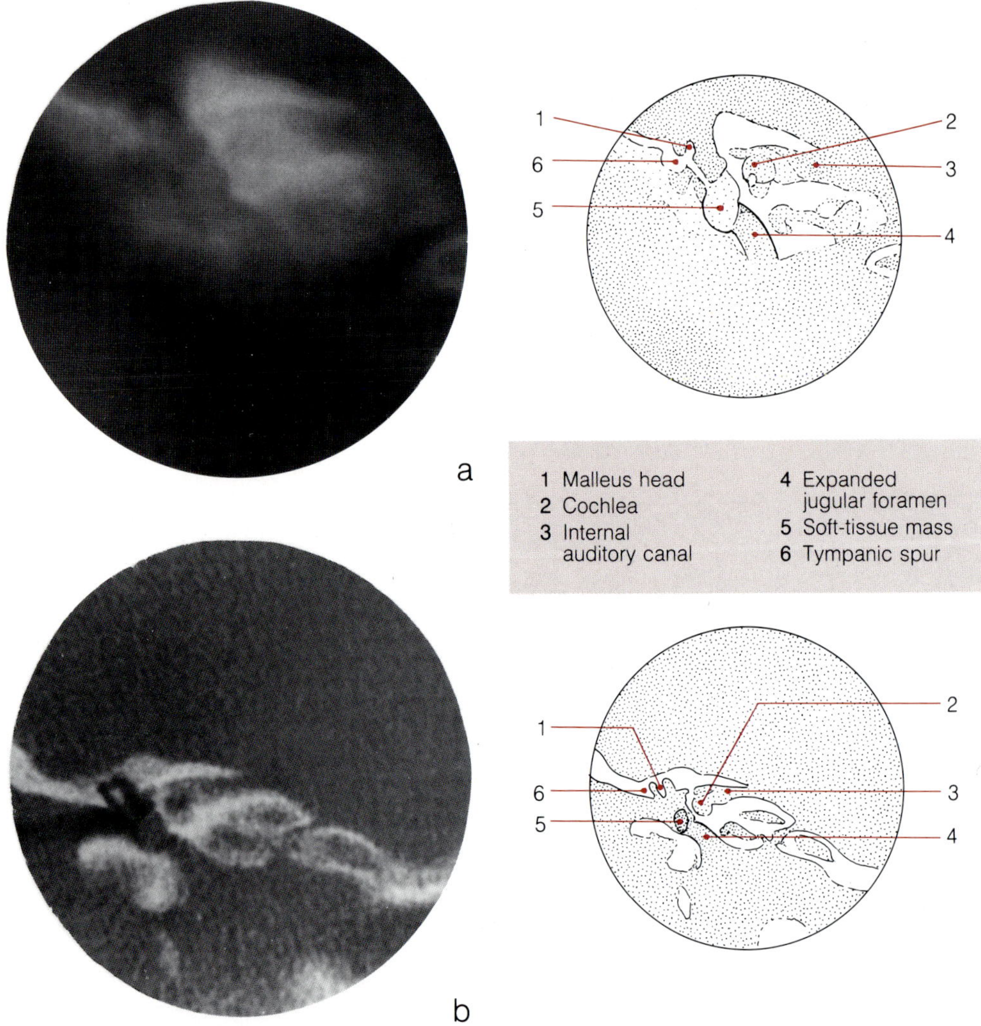

Fig. 1.11 Glomus jugulare tumor. *a* Coronal complex-motion tomographic cut and *b* high-resolution CT scan at the same anatomic plane show a soft-tissue mass arising in the region of the jugular foramen and extending into the middle-ear cleft. While bone detail is exquisite on the complex-motion tomogram, it is equally sharp on the CT scan; however, the CT scan shows the soft-tissue mass much more clearly. (Courtesy of C. Guirado, MD, Barcelona, Spain.)

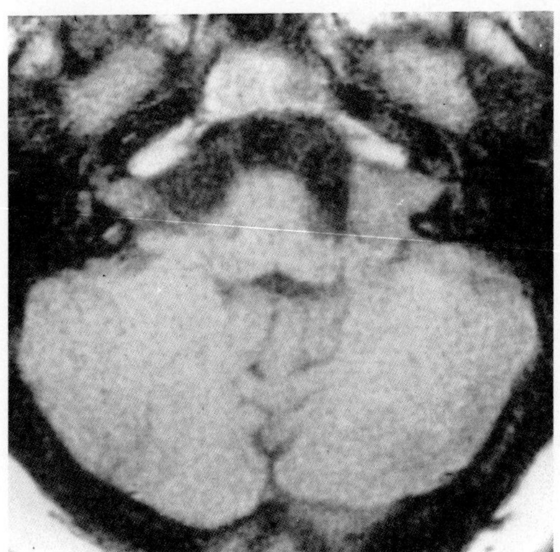

Fig. 1.12 Bilateral acoustic neuromas demonstrated by magnetic resonance imaging (MRI). *This man with neurofibromatosis presented with bilateral sensorineural hearing loss. Axial projection of a T2-weighted MRI scan performed on a 1.5 tesla scanner shows bilateral intracanalicular eighth nerve tumors (acoustic neuromas). On the left, the tumor widens the porus acousticus and extends into the cerebropontine angle. On the right, the tumor barely protrudes into the porus acousticus. (Courtesy of D. Chakares, MD, Columbus, Ohio.)*

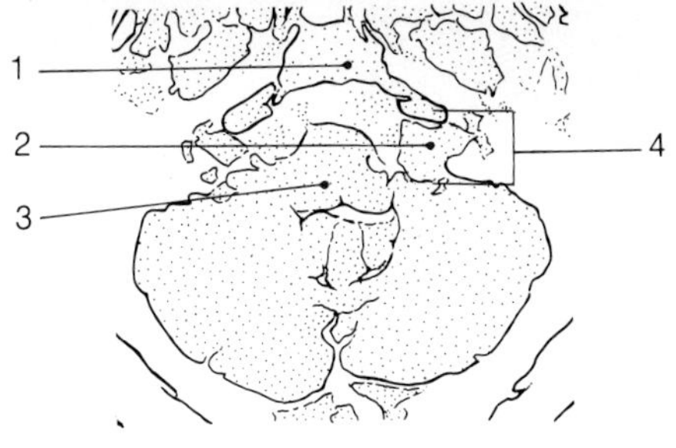

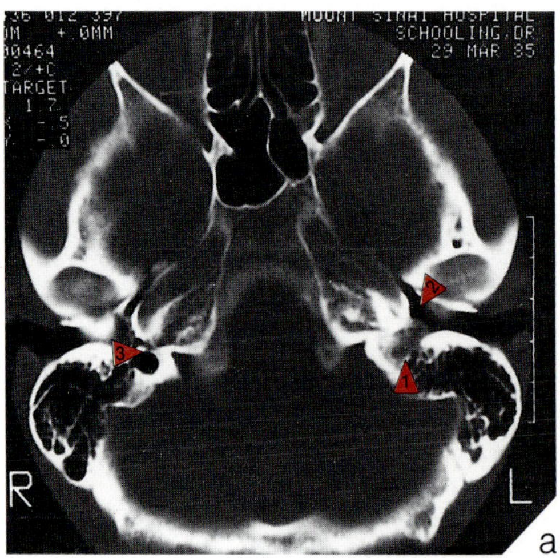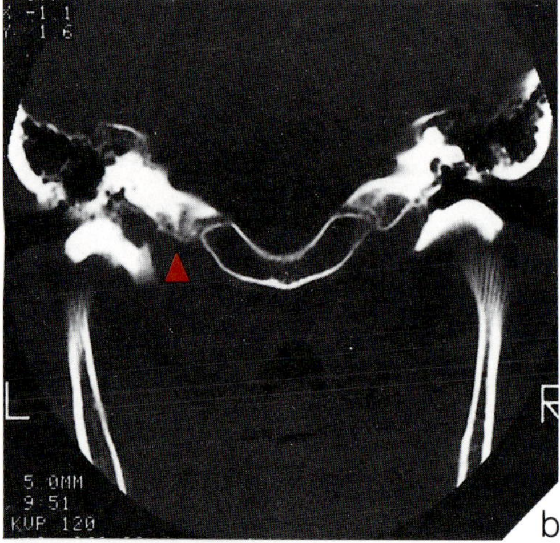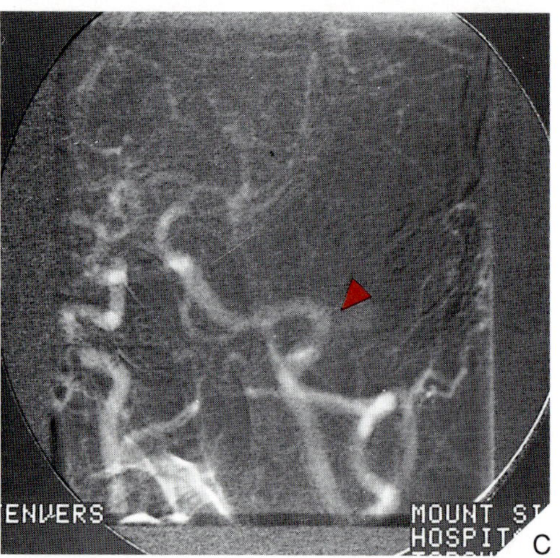

Fig. 1.13 Intraarterial embolization of glomus jugulare tumor. *a An axial high-resolution CT scan in a 46-year-old man shows bone destruction (arrow 1) in the region of the left jugular bulb with a soft-tissue mass (arrow 2). The normal jugular foramen (arrow 3) is also shown. b Coronal scan (bone window) shows bone expansion and destruction (arrow) in the region of the left jugular bulb. c Digital subtraction angiogram (DSA) demonstrates the vascular blush of the glomus jugulare tumor (arrow). d Selective arteriogram shows that the tumor is supplied primarily by the ascending pharyngeal artery (arrow). e Repeat arteriogram following partial embolization of the tumor with polyvinyl alcohol microspheres shows a marked decrease in the size of the vascular stain. f At the end of the embolization procedure only a minute vascular stain remains. The subsequent surgical procedure was almost bloodless.*

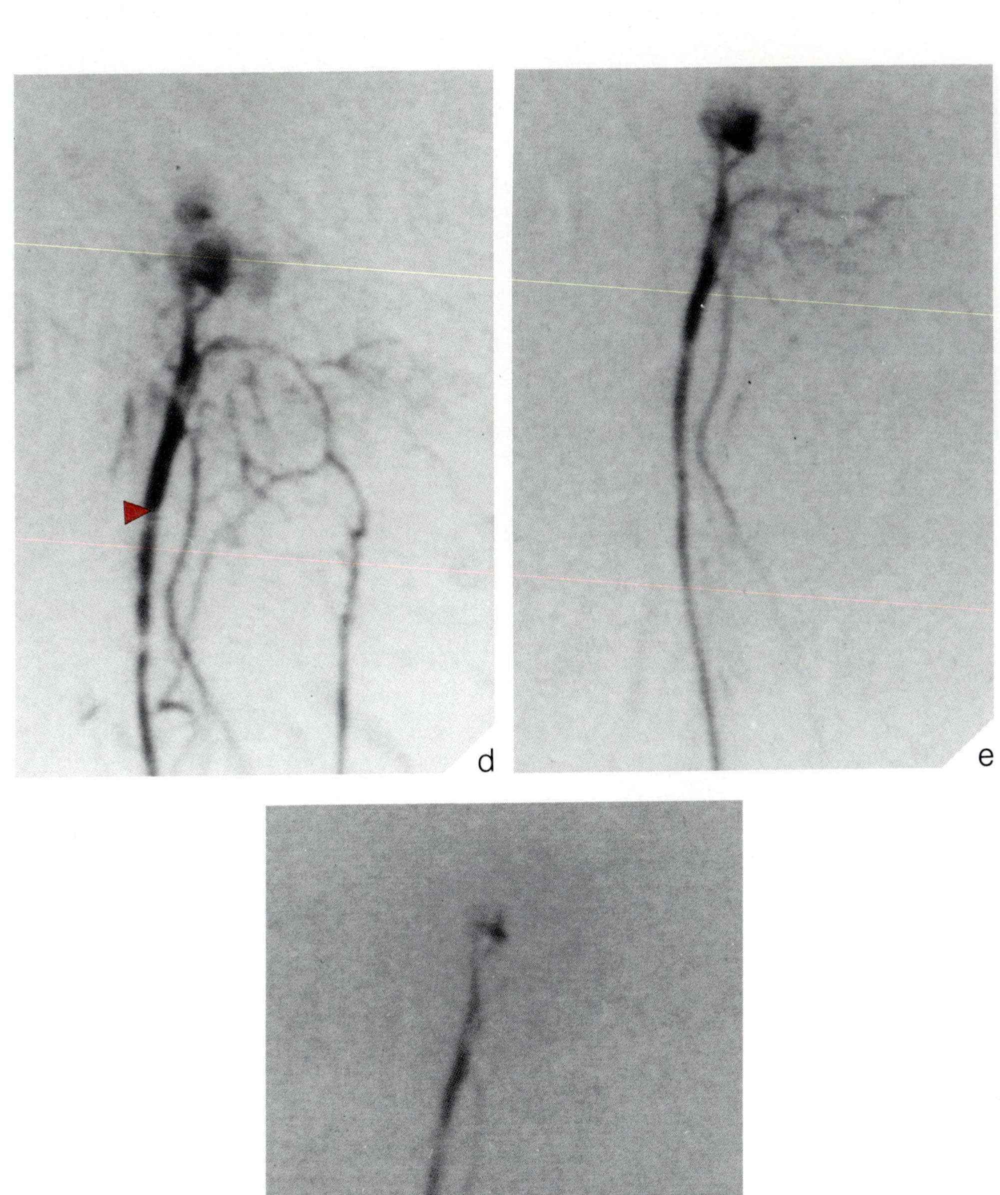

d
e
f

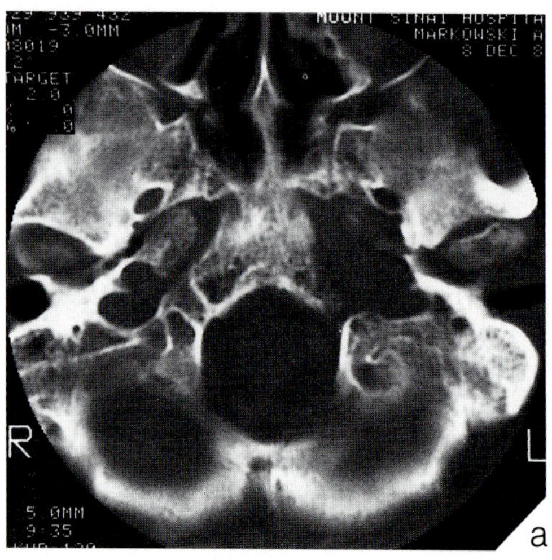

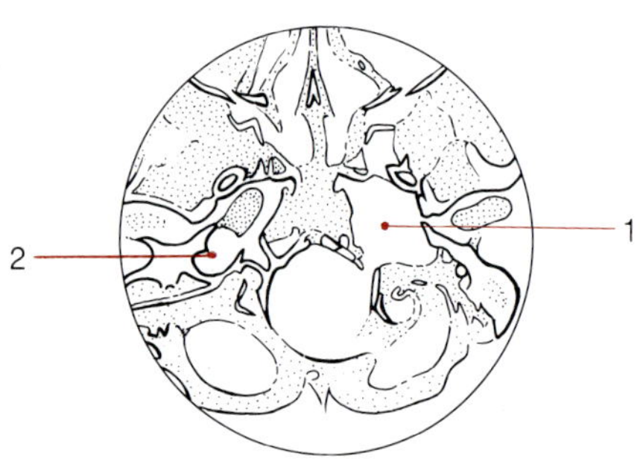

1 Destruction		**3** Decreased uptake	
2 Normal jugular foramen		**4** Increased uptake	

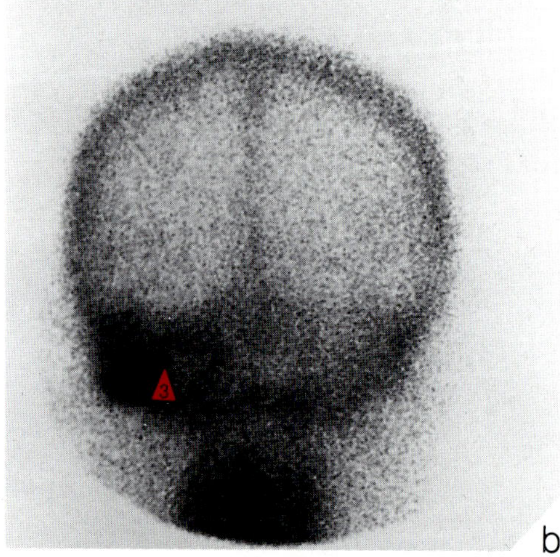

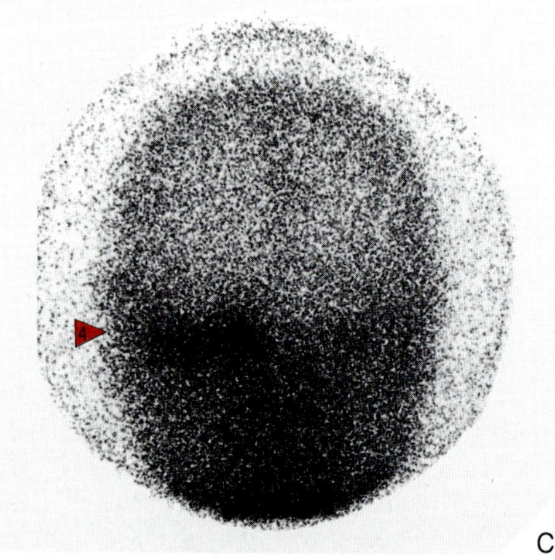

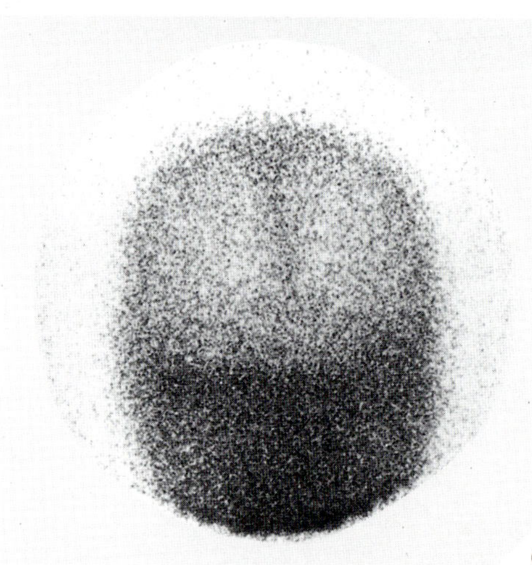

Fig. 1.14 Osteomyelitis of the temporal bone.
a A high-resolution CT scan (axial projection) at the level of the skull base shows widespread destruction in the region of the left jugular foramen. Note loss of cortical definition at the margin of the bony defect. Compare with the normal jugular foramen. b The delayed phase of a methylene diphosphonate (MDP) bone scan (posterior view) shows increased uptake throughout the left temporal bone indicating increased osteoblastic activity. The region of decreased uptake (arrow 3) within the "hot" zone presumably represents necrotic bone. c Prior to treatment, the gallium citrate scan (posterior view) shows increased uptake (arrow 4) throughout the temporal bone. d Following successful antibiotic treatment, the gallium scan (posterior view) is normal. (Reproduced with permission from Noyek, 1984.)

Paranasal Sinuses

Except for interventional endoscopic methods, the paranasal sinuses are virtually inaccessible to direct clinical evaluation. Radiographic examinations of the paranasal sinuses account for more than half the radiologic imaging studies in otolaryngology–head and neck surgery. The radiographic hallmarks of sinus disease are: (1) altered air content; (2) thickening of the lining (mucous membrane); and (3) involvement of adjacent bony structures. In general, diseases of the paranasal sinuses, as well as certain congenital malformations and anatomic variants, are perceived radiographically as an increase or decrease in transradiancy ("density") of the affected sinus. One or more sinuses may be affected, and involvement of an affected sinus may be focal or diffuse. The specific radiologic signs of paranasal sinus disease are tabulated in Figure 2.1.

A thorough plain film examination usually suffices for diagnosis and management in patients with acute infective sinusitis (Figs. 2.2, 2.3). Periapical films and/or panoramic tomography may demonstrate underlying dental pathology in patients with maxillary sinusitis (Fig. 2.4). Chronic mucosal hypertrophy, mucous-retention cysts, and polyps are common in patients with respiratory allergies, and can be demonstrated by plain films (Fig. 2.5) or by more sophisticated techniques. Figure 2.6 demonstrates cystic masses both on a Water's view and on a CT scan. Magnetic resonance imaging can also be used in the examination of cysts (Fig. 2.7). Osteomas of the sinuses are not uncommon and are easily diagnosed by conventional radiographic techniques (Fig. 2.8).

Opacification of a paranasal sinus is a nonspecific finding: it may indicate the presence of thickened mucosa, pus, blood, serous effusion, cerebrospinal fluid, or neoplasm. High-resolution ultrasound, CT, or MRI may be very informative in

FIG. 2.1 RADIOLOGIC SIGNS OF PARANASAL SINUS DISEASE.

Decreased aeration (luminal opacification)	Changes in bony walls
Mucosal thickening	Demineralization
Air–fluid level	Osteolysis
Cyst formation	Dehiscence
Soft-tissue mass	Fracture
Emphysema	Sclerosis (osteoblastosis)
Calcification	Sequestrum
Ossification	Thickening
Foreign body (bodies)	Displacement
Teeth (embryonic or adult)	Reduction in sinus cavity volume

such cases (Figs. 2.9, 2.10). The CT findings are pathognomonic in patients with rhinoliths of the nasal cavity (Fig. 2.11).

It is important to demonstrate (or exclude) intraorbital and/or intracranial extension of disease in patients with complicated infections, mucoceles, or neoplastic disease. Although complex-motion tomography accurately depicts bone destruction, soft-tissue abnormalities are poorly defined by this technique. Soft-tissue abnormalities (Figs. 2.12–2.15) can be clearly demonstrated using high-resolution CT. This technique is well

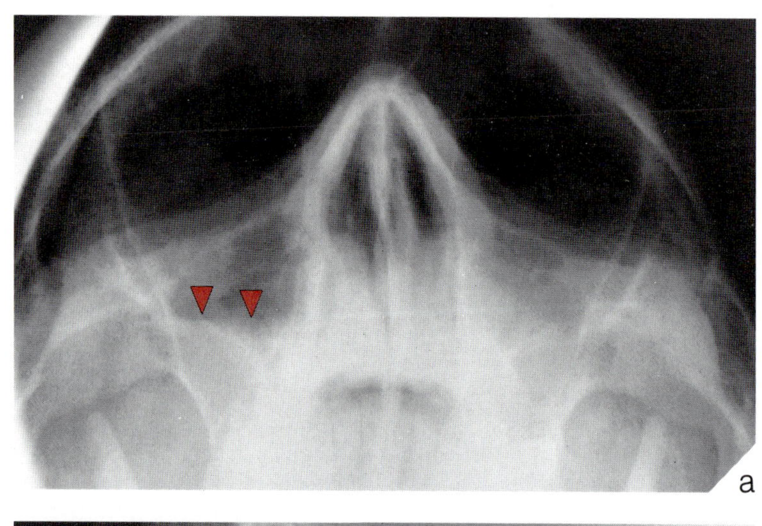

a

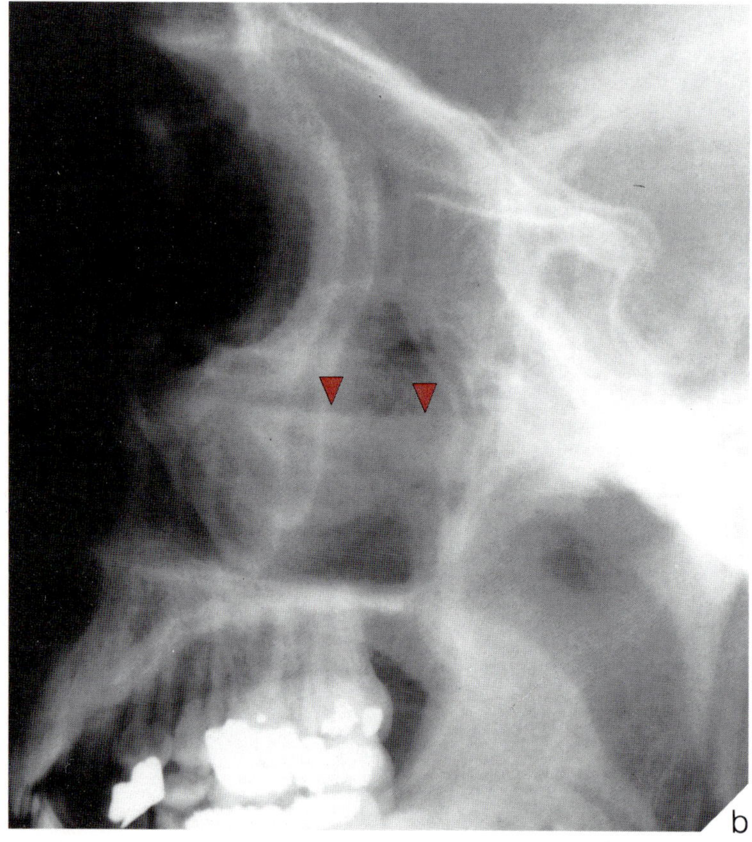

b

suited for the visualization of bone destruction associated with soft-tissue abnormalities (Figs. 2.12, 2.16), and is indispensable in the pretreatment staging of malignant neoplasms (Figs. 2.17–2.19). MRI provides a high-resolution planar display of soft-tissue structures comparable to that seen on CT. Because calcium is invisible on MRI scans (see Fig. 2.7), bone destruction cannot be detected by this modality. Angiography, radionuclide bone scans, or gallium scintigraphy may provide important information in selected cases (Figs. 2.19, 2.20).

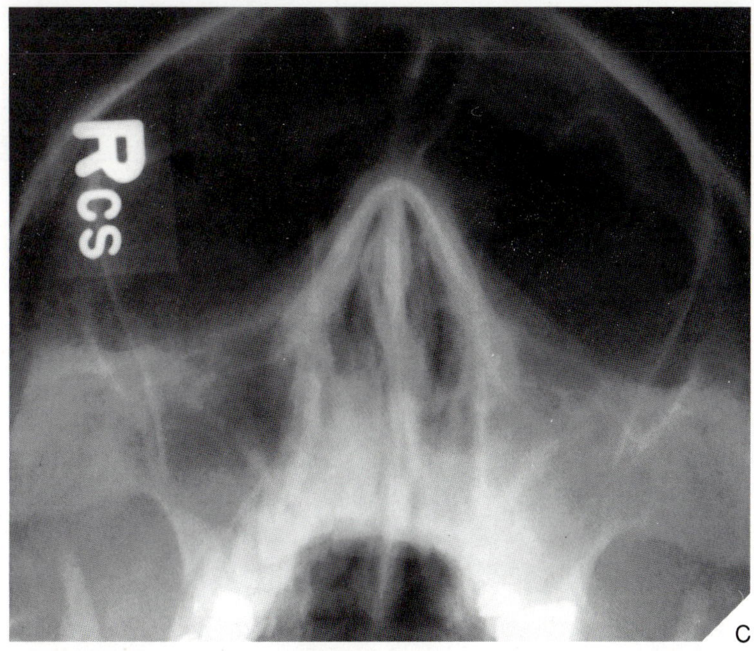

C

Fig. 2.2 Acute purulent sinusitis of the right maxillary sinus and mucosal thickening of the left maxillary sinus. *A 24-year-old man with symptoms of acute sinusitis.* ***a*** *A Waters projection shows an air–fluid level (arrows) in the right maxillary sinus and complete opacification of the left maxillary sinus.* ***b*** *The lateral projection shows opacification of the ethmoid labyrinth and sphenoid sinuses, as well as an air–fluid level (arrows) in the right maxillary sinus.* ***c*** *Following antibiotic therapy, the right maxillary sinus is fully aerated. The left maxillary sinus remains opacified, presumably due to thickened mucosa. (Note: It is not possible to tell from plain films or conventional tomograms whether sinus opacification is due to mucosal thickening or to fluid.)*

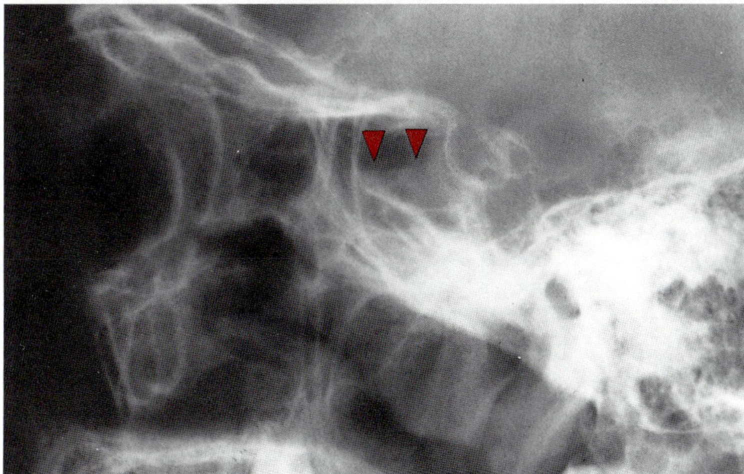

Fig. 2.3 Acute purulent sphenoiditis. *An 18-year-old man with acute sinusitis. A lateral radiograph shows air–fluid levels in the sphenoid sinuses (arrows). (Reproduced with permission from Noyek, Wortzman, Kassel, 1987.)*

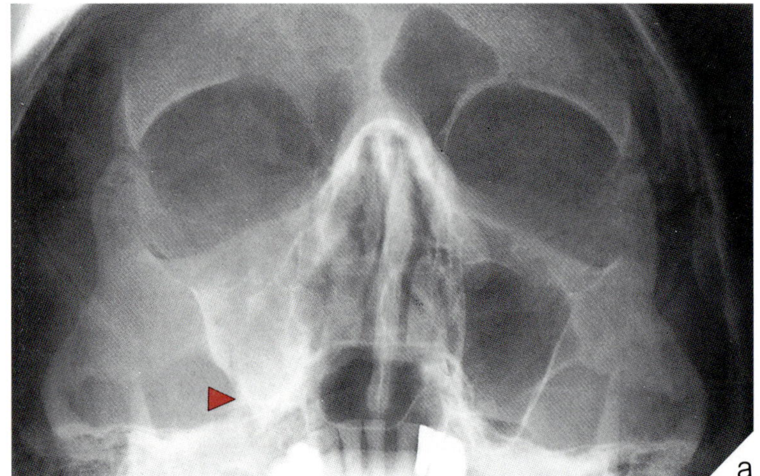

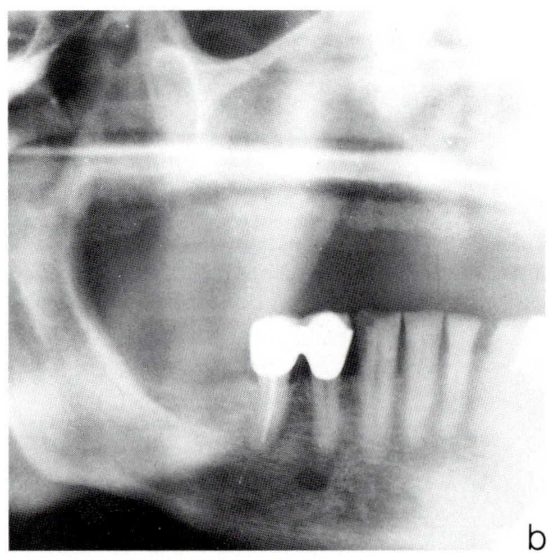

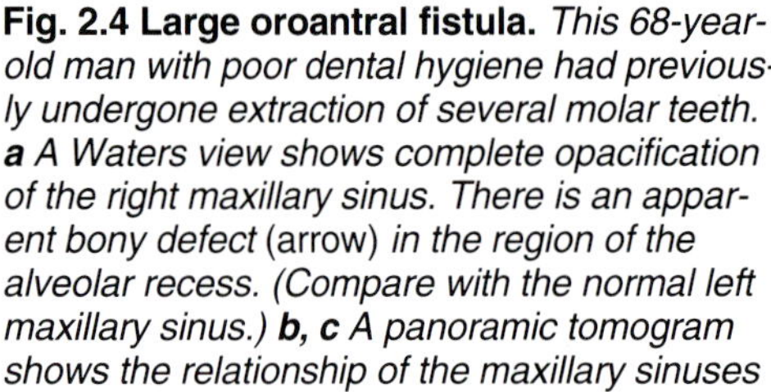

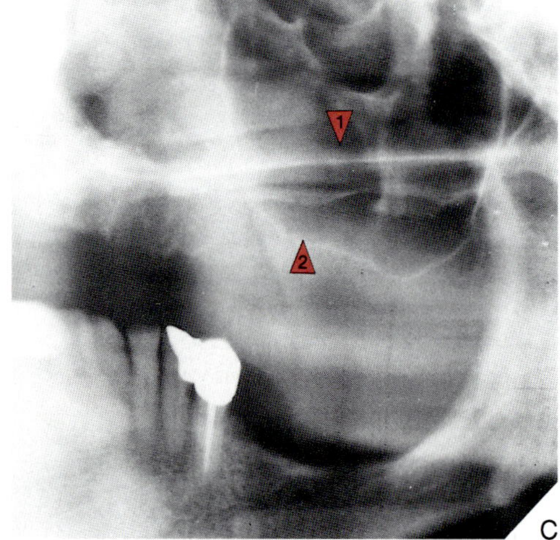

Fig. 2.4 Large oroantral fistula. *This 68-year-old man with poor dental hygiene had previously undergone extraction of several molar teeth. **a** A Waters view shows complete opacification of the right maxillary sinus. There is an apparent bony defect (arrow) in the region of the alveolar recess. (Compare with the normal left maxillary sinus.) **b, c** A panoramic tomogram shows the relationship of the maxillary sinuses to the supporting structures. **b** The right maxillary sinus is opaque. The alveolar process cannot be identified. Destruction of the inferior wall of the maxillary sinus and adjacent maxilla has created a large oroantral fistula. **c** The normal left maxillary sinus is shown for comparison. All of the maxillary teeth are absent bilaterally. The floor of the nasal cavity is indicated (arrow 1) as is the alveolar recess (arrow 2).*

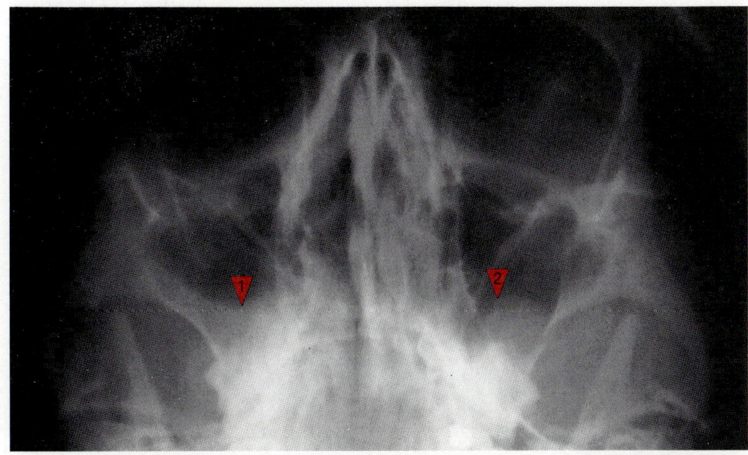

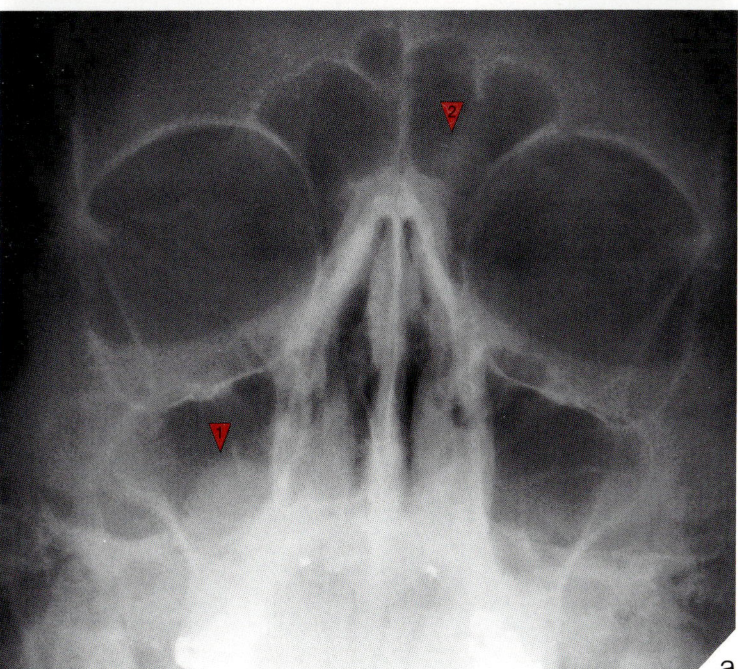

a

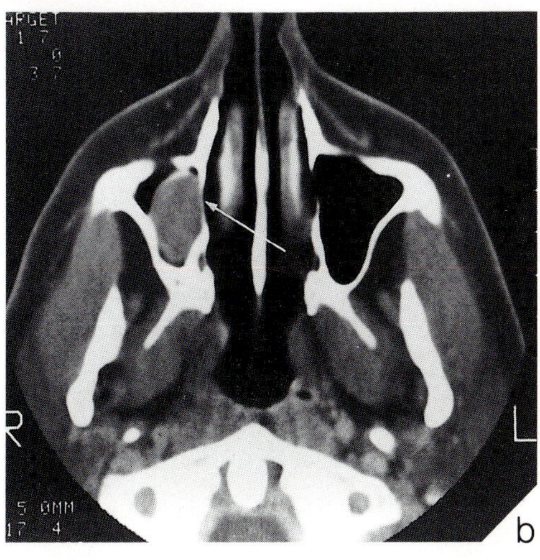

b

Fig. 2.5 Air–fluid level In the right maxillary sinus; retention cyst in the left maxillary sinus. *A Waters view in a 26-year-old woman demonstrates an air–fluid level in the right maxillary sinus. Note upward slope of fluid level in zygomatic recess (rising meniscus) (arrow 1). A dome-shaped retention cyst (arrow 2) occupies the lower third of the left maxillary sinus. This is a typical location for these innocent lesions, which contain serous fluid or mucus and do not destroy bone. (Reproduced with permission from Noyek, Wortzman, Kassel, 1987.)*

Fig. 2.6 Multiple retention cysts. *a A Waters view in a 35-year-old man demonstrates a dome-shaped cystic mass profiled by air in the lower half of the right maxillary sinus (arrow 1). A similar lesion is seen in the lower portion of the left frontal sinus (arrow 2). b A CT scan (axial plane) demonstrates a homogeneous oval cystic mass abutting the medial wall of the maxillary sinus. There is no evidence of bone destruction.*

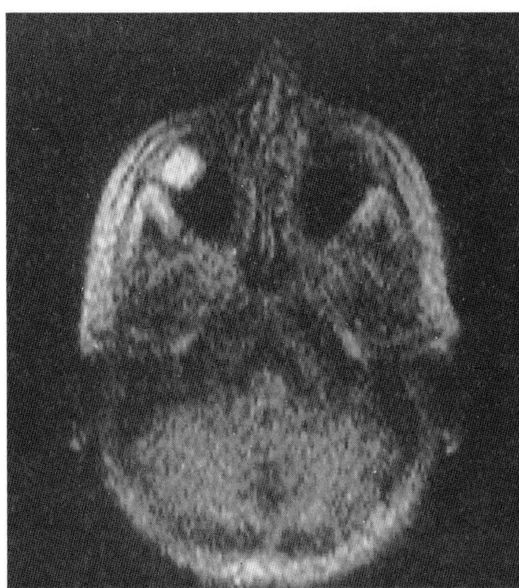

Fig. 2.7 Retention cyst. *A T2-weighted MRI (axial plane) shows a mucous retention cyst in the anterolateral portion of the right maxillary sinus. Bone cannot be imaged by MRI; hence the wall of the maxillary sinus is invisible (compare Fig. 2.6b). Stagnant fluid collections (e.g., cyst contents) appear white on T2-weighted scans, which are noisier and have less resolution than T1-weighted scans.*

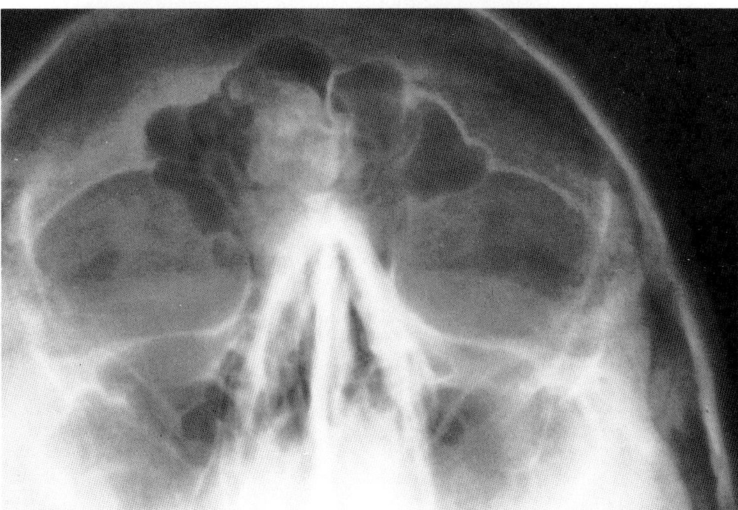

Fig. 2.8 Osteoma of frontal sinus. *A Waters view demonstrates a bony mass in the right frontal sinus. The superior and lateral margins of the mass are sharply profiled by air. The osteoma, which contains both cortical and cancellous bone, encroaches on the left frontal sinus. This was an incidental finding in a 62-year-old man with symptoms of maxillary sinusitis.*

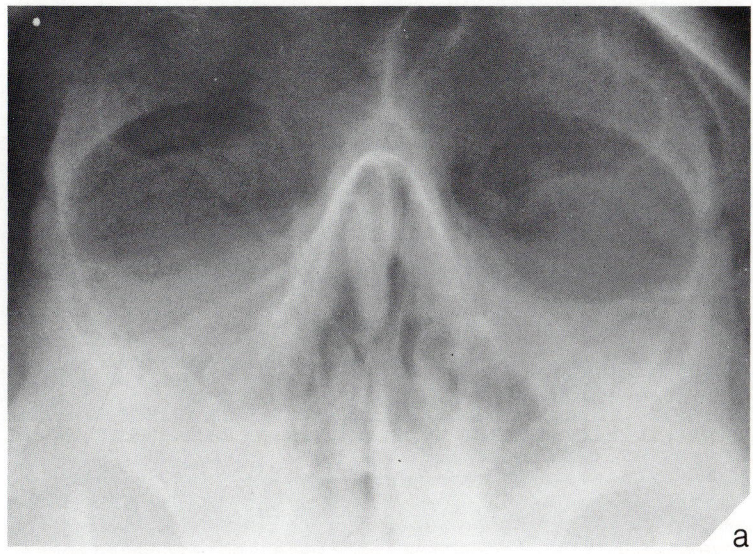

Fig. 2.9 Chronic purulent maxillary sinusitis. *This 59-year-old woman had a history of recurrent episodes of maxillary sinusitis. **a** A Waters projection demonstrates opacification of the right maxillary sinus, which is presumably filled with pus and thickened mucosa. There is marked mucosal thickening in the left maxillary sinus, but some air is present. **b** A transverse high-resolution sonogram (sector scan) of the right maxillary sinus shows that it is filled with echogenic material (arrow 1). The back wall of the maxillary sinus (arrow 2) is sharply defined, indicating that the sinus is filled with fluid. **c** A comparable image of the left maxillary sinus fails to demonstrate the posterior wall due to acoustic shadowing by air in the sinus cavity. (Note: The ultrasonic pulse is almost completely attenuated by air; therefore structures deep to an air collection cannot be imaged. Ultrasound can differentiate fluid from solid tissue when the maxillary or frontal sinus is completely opacified, but is likely to be uninformative if the sinus is not completely opacified, i.e., if any residual air is present.)*

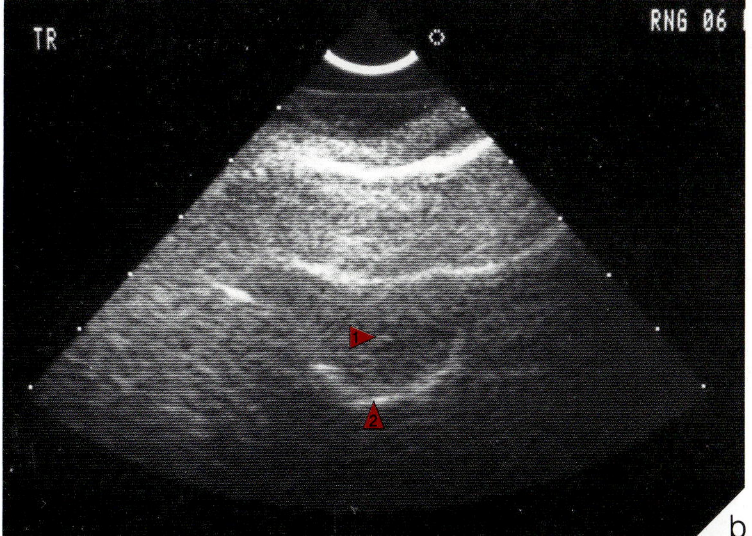

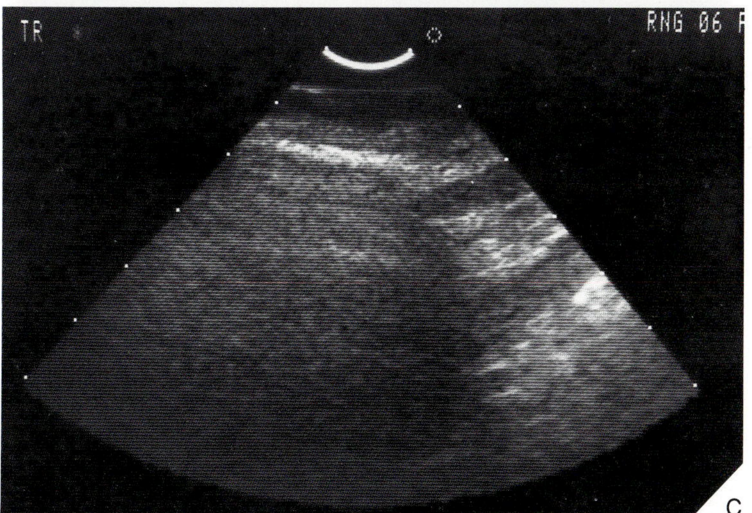

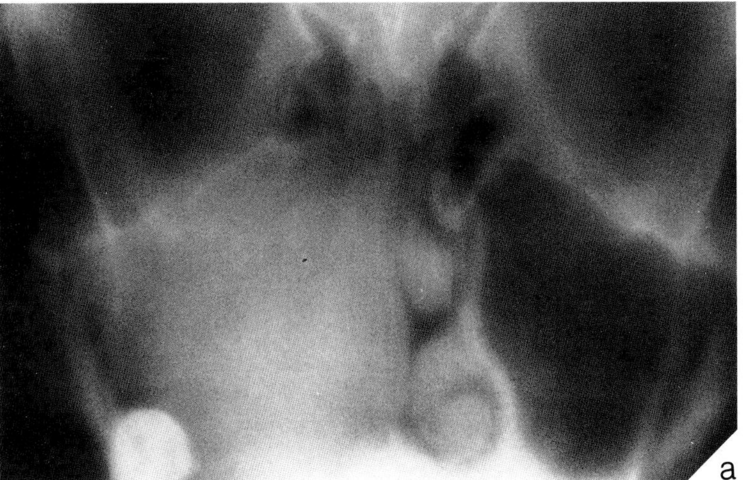

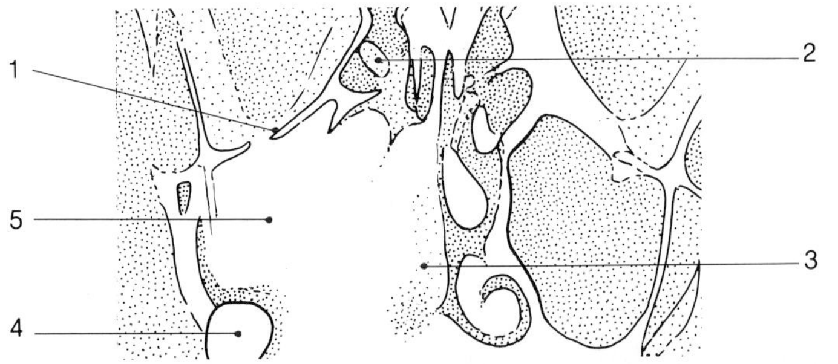

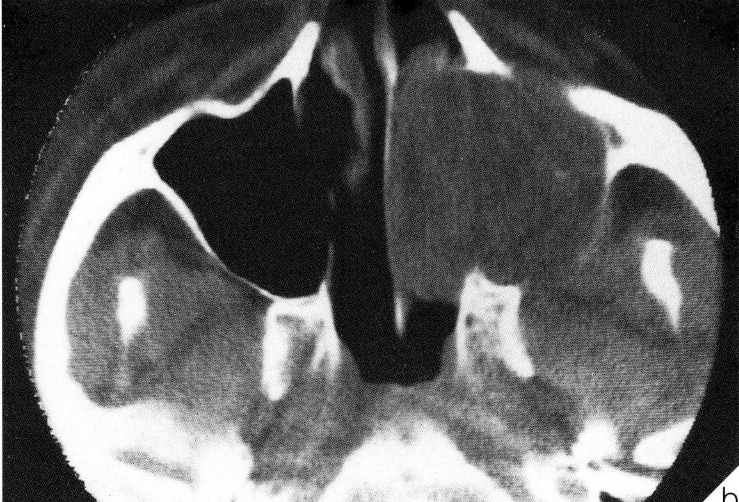

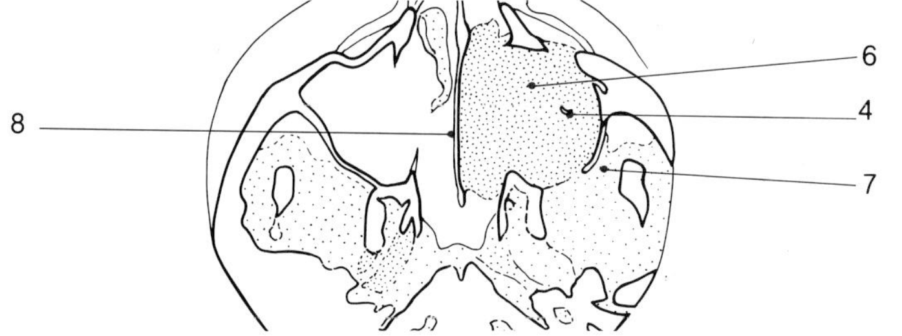

Fig. 2.10 Dentigerous cyst of the maxillary sinus. *This 32-year-old man presented with sinusitis and a nasal discharge. **a** A complex-motion tomogram (coronal projection) shows a huge expansile mass within the right maxillary sinus. The medial wall of the right maxillary sinus has been destroyed and the mass fills the nasal cavity on this side. The floor of the orbit is intact. Although it is not possible to say whether the mass is cystic or solid, the presence of a tooth within the lesion suggests that it is a dentigerous cyst. **b** An axial CT scan demonstrates a soft-tissue mass in the right maxillary sinus and right nasal cavity. The posterior wall of the maxillary sinus is bowed outward and thinned. The medial wall of the sinus has been destroyed. The mass fills the right nasal cavity, extending posteriorly nearly to the level of the choana. The small calcific density within the mass probably represents the tooth, which is not completely included in this cut.*

1 Floor of right orbit
2 Uninvolved ethmoid cells
3 Opacified right nasal cavity
4 Tooth
5 Opacified maxillary sinus
6 Cystic mass expanding right maxillary sinus
7 Displaced posterior wall of right maxillary sinus
8 Displaced nasal septum

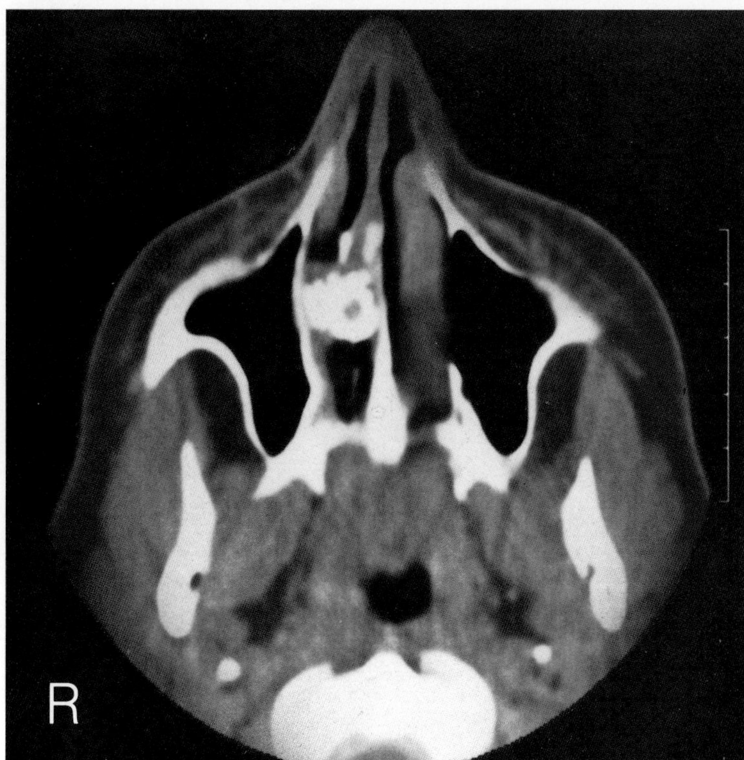

Fig. 2.11 Rhinolith. *Axial CT cut demonstrates a heavily calcified mass in the midportion of the right nasal cavity. The mass (rhinolith) is covered anteriorly by thickened mucosa. The nasal septum is intact.*

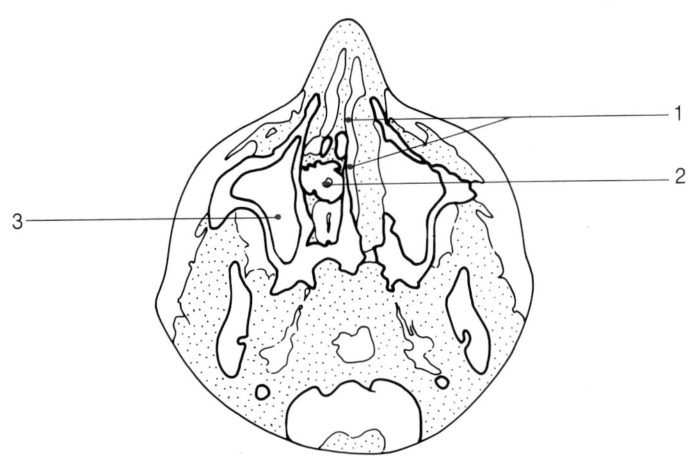

1 Nasal septum	**3** Right maxillary sinus
2 Rhinolith	

**Fig. 2.12 Frontoethmoid muco-
cele.** *This 48-year-old man presented with left-side proptosis. **a** A
Caldwell view demonstrates a discrete expansile mass (arrows 4)
that encroaches on the central portion of both frontal sinuses, as well
as a soft-tissue density within the
left ethmoid labyrinth. The lamina
papyracea between the left eth-
moidal labyrinth and the orbit
appears to be intact. **b** A complex-
motion tomogram shows that the
mass (mucocele) has eroded the
superior margin of the frontal sinus
(arrows 1). There is loss of bone in
the superomedial aspect of the left
orbit (arrow 2). **c** A coronal CT
scan shows a soft-tissue mass in
the medial portion of the orbit
which is displacing the globe laterally (compare with normal right
orbit). The left ethmoid labyrinth,
where the mucocele originated,
has been obliterated. Several ethmoid cells are opacified on the
right, but there is no discrete mass.
d An axial CT scan demonstrates
the relations between the ethmoid
mucocele (arrow 7) and the left
orbit. The wall of the posterior ethmoid labyrinth is displaced posteriorly (arrow 8). The left globe is displaced anteriorly and laterally, and
bone destruction is evident anteriorly. **e** A coronal cut (anterior to the
plane shown in **c**) shows extensive
bone destruction (arrow 9) over the
superior aspect of the mucocele
(arrow 4), which could allow it to
extend intracranially. The ethmoid
mucocele has displaced the thin
orbital wall inferiorly and laterally
(arrow 10).*

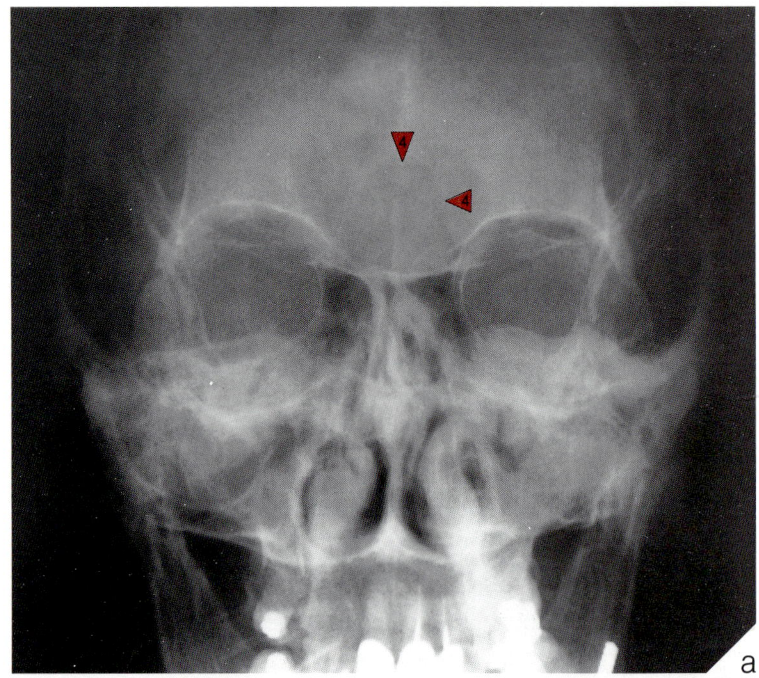

a

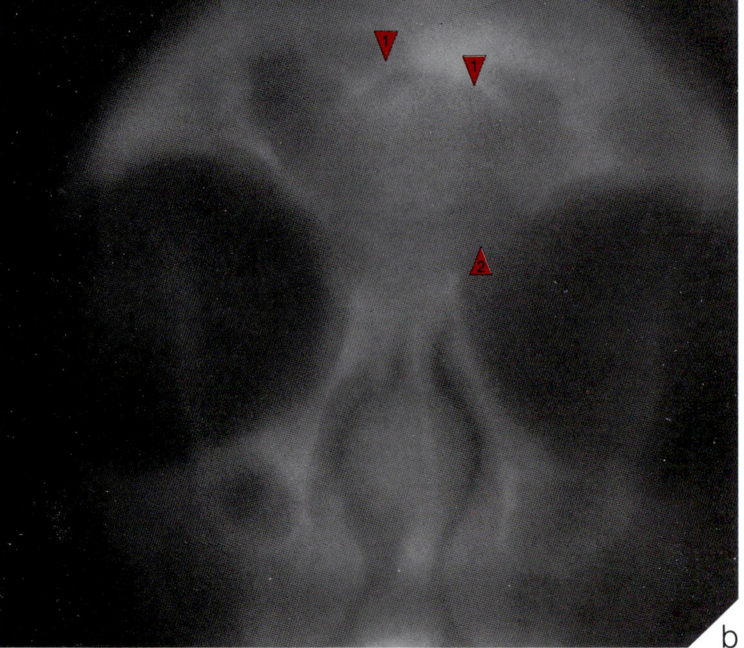

b

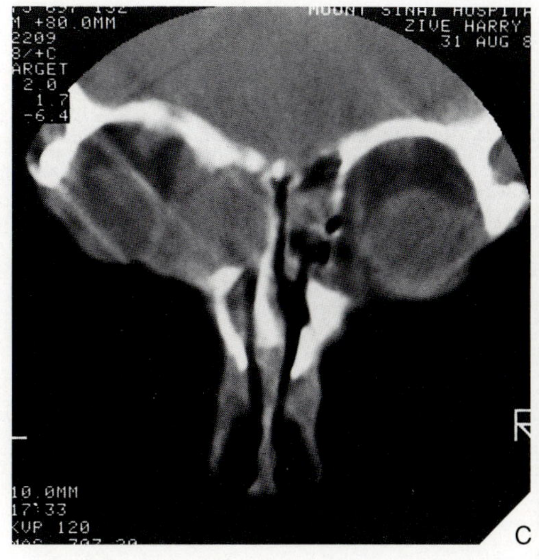

c

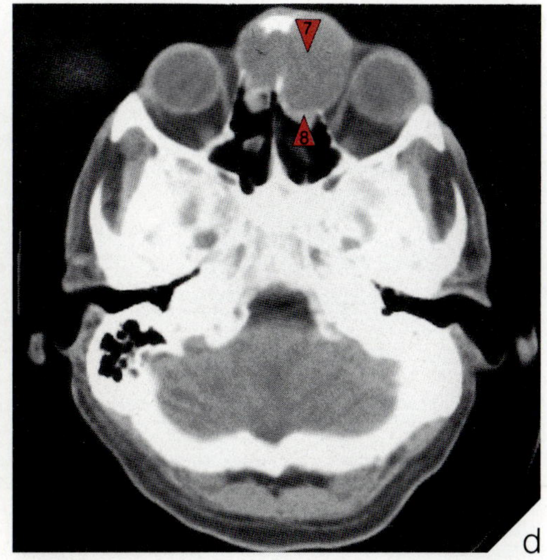

d

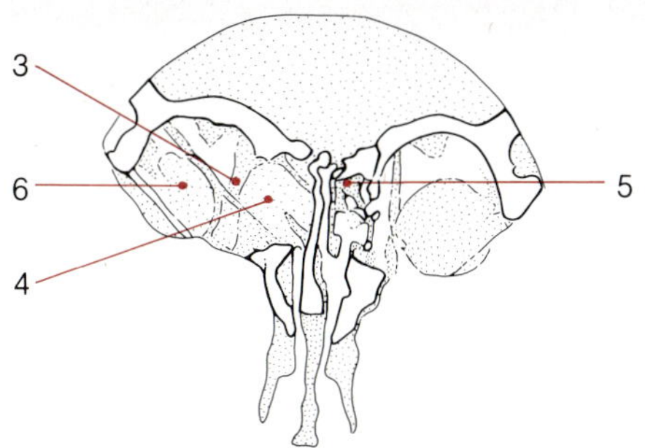

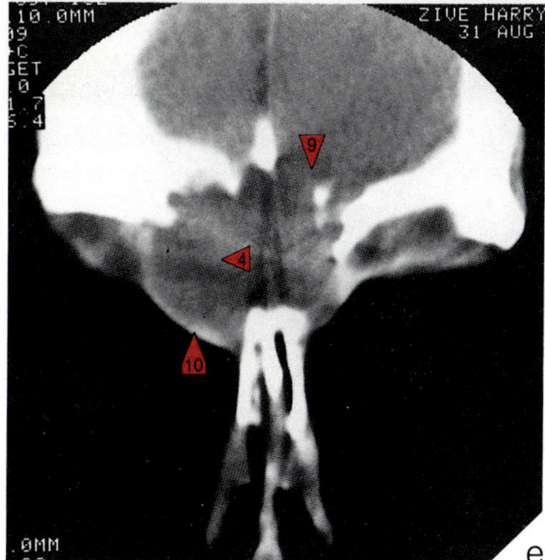

e

1 Eroded superior margin of frontal sinus	**6** Proptosed globe
2 Superomedial aspect of left orbit	**7** Ethmoid mucocele
3 Margins of mucocele	**8** Wall of posterior ethmoid labyrinth
4 Mucocele	**9** Bone destruction
5 Thickened mucous membrane in right ethmoid labyrinth	**10** Orbital wall displacement

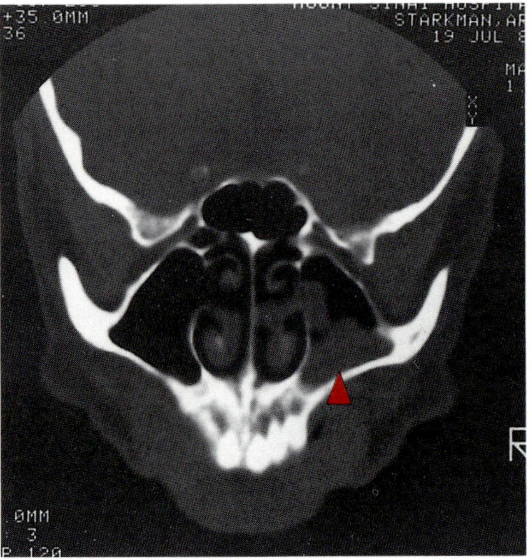

Fig. 2.13 Inverting papilloma of the maxillary sinus. *A coronal CT scan in a 66-year-old man shows a lobulated tumor* (arrow) *sharply profiled by air in the inferior and medial portion of the right maxillary sinus. The tumor has extended into the nasal cavity via the middle meatus. There is no bone destruction.*

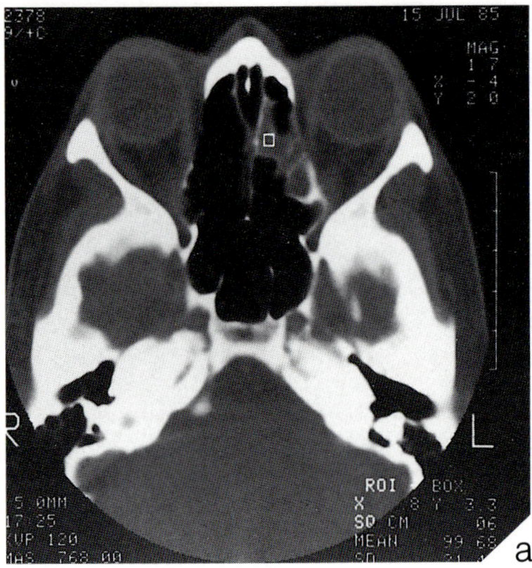

a

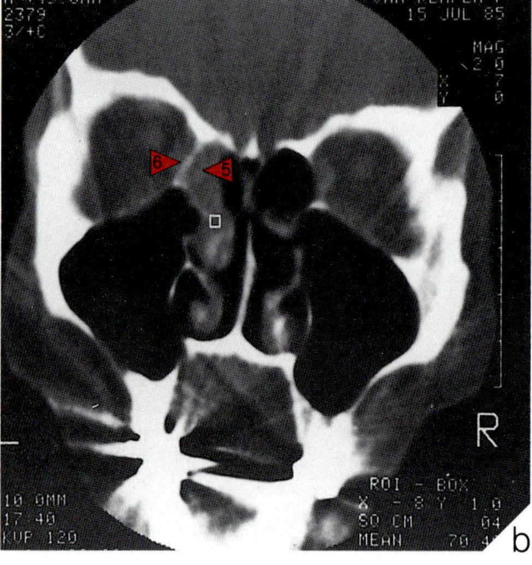

b

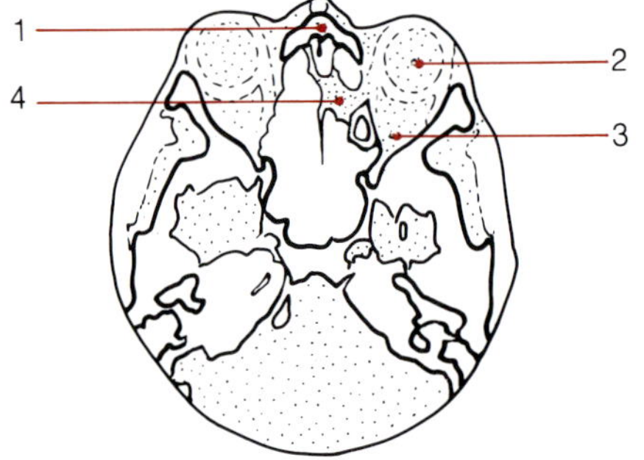

1 Nasal bones	5 Tumor
2 Left eyeball	6 Lamina
3 Orbital apex	papyracea
4 Opacified left ethmoid cleft	

Fig. 2.14 Inverting papilloma of the ethmoid sinus. *This 47-year-old woman presented with what appeared on physical examination to be a single nasal polyp. **a** An axial CT scan demonstrates mucosal thickening in the region of the left ethmoid labyrinth* (cursor) *and opacification of a posterior ethmoid cell. There is no bone destruction. **b** A coronal CT scan defines the relationships of the ethmoid tumor more precisely. The tumor* (arrow 5) *abuts the medial orbital wall and the superomedial wall of the maxillary sinus. The lamina papyracea* (arrow 6) *between the ethmoid labyrinth and the left orbit, as well as the roof of the ethmoid labyrinth, are intact. The maxillary sinus is uninvolved. (The cursor is positioned over the attachment of the left middle turbinate.)*

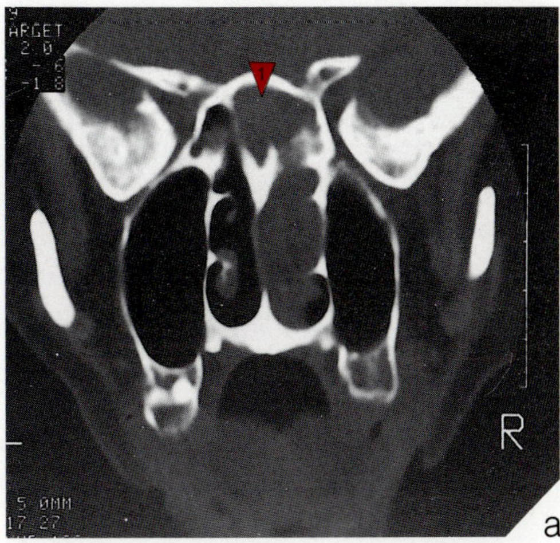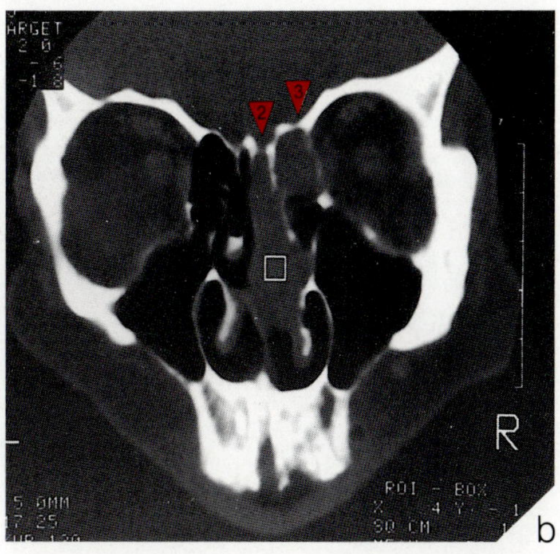

Fig. 2.15 Inverting papilloma of the nasal cavity and sphenoid sinus. *This 70-year-old woman presented with nasal obstruction.*
a Coronal CT scan through the posterior portion of the nasal cavity demonstrates a soft-tissue mass (arrow 1) in the right nasal cavity which is markedly expanded. The right sphe- *noid sinus is opacified; whether this represents tumor or retained secretions cannot be ascertained. b On a more anterior coronal cut the cursor is positioned over the nasal mass. The right cribriform plate (arrow 2) and the roof of the ethmoid labyrinth (arrow 3) are intact.*

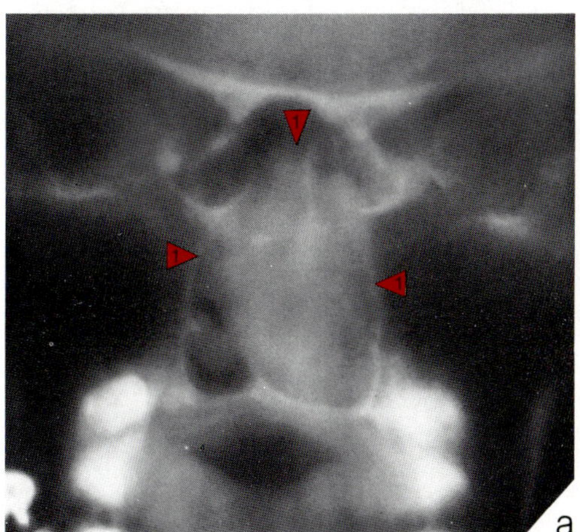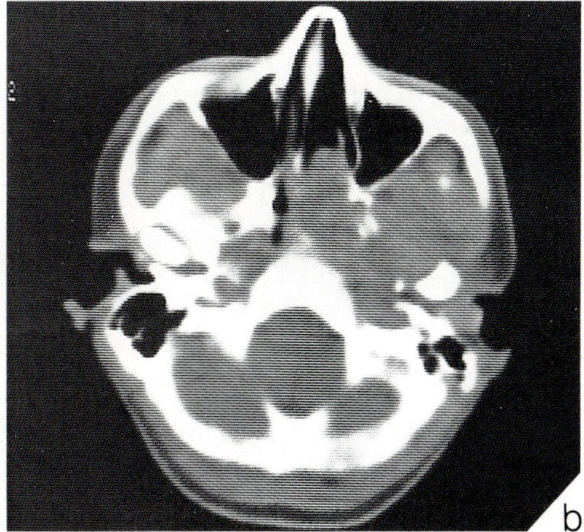

Fig. 2.16 Nasopharyngeal angiofibroma. *A 16-year-old boy presented with a massive epistaxis. a A complex-motion coronal tomogram shows marked expansion of the left nasal cavity, containing a large soft-tissue mass, an angiofibroma (arrows 1). The tumor, originating in the nasopharynx, extends cephalad into the sphenoid sinus. b An axial CT scan shows the tumor's soft-tissue relationships, and its propensity to destroy contiguous bony structures. Anteriorly the tumor extends into the left nasal cavity. Posterolaterally it has destroyed the medial aspect of the pterygoid process. An intact fascial plane separates the tumor from the muscular structures of the infratemporal fossa. The external pterygoid muscle, which runs between the lateral pterygoid plate and the mandibular condyle, is free of tumor.*

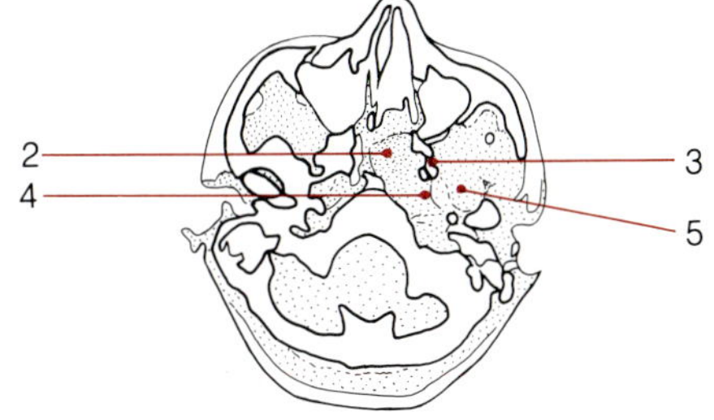

1 Angiofibroma	4 Intact fascial planes
2 Tumor	
3 Bone destruction	5 Intact external pterygoid muscle

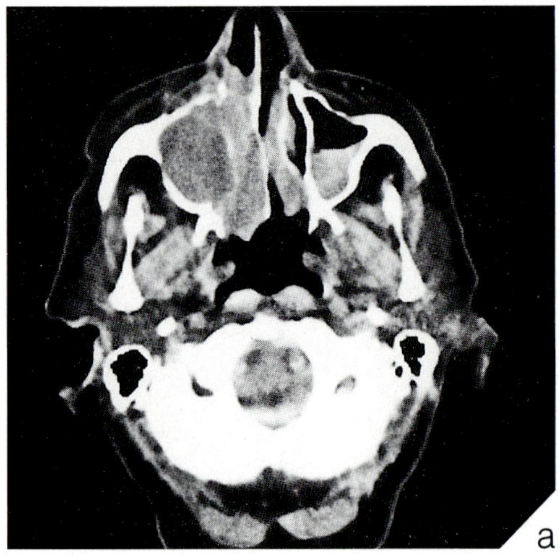

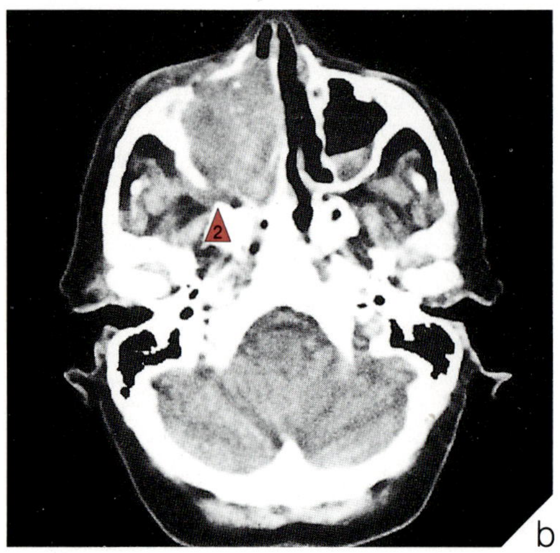

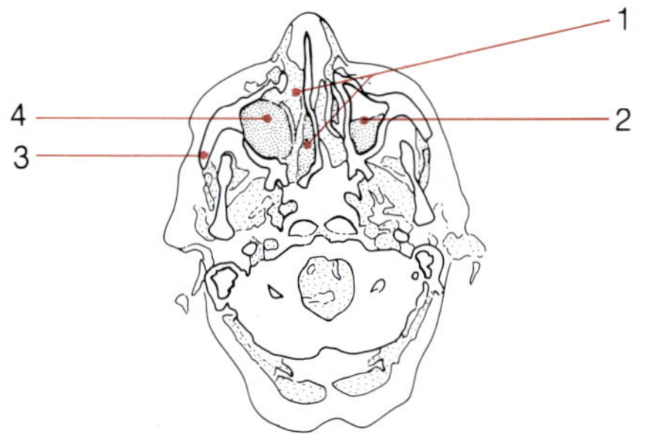

1 Tumor in nasal cavity
2 Air-blood level
3 Bone destruction
4 Necrotic portion of tumor in maxillary sinus

Fig. 2.17. Squamous cell carcinoma of the maxillary sinus. *a* An axial CT scan demonstrates a large expansile mass within the right maxillary sinus of a 77-year-old woman. The tumor completely fills the right maxillary sinus. The medial wall of the maxillary sinus is disrupted and the tumor extends anteriorly and posteriorly into the right nasal cavity. There is also a localized area of bone destruction in the posterolateral wall of the maxillary sinus. A portion of the tumor is necrotic, as indicated by its decreased attenuation (density). The left maxillary sinus contains an air–blood level. *b* An axial cut at the level of the zygomatic arches shows obvious bone destruction both anteriorly and posteriorly (arrow 2). The fat plane marginating the posterior wall of the right maxillary sinus is obliterated, indicating extension of tumor into the temporal fossa. Compare with intact at plane on opposite side.

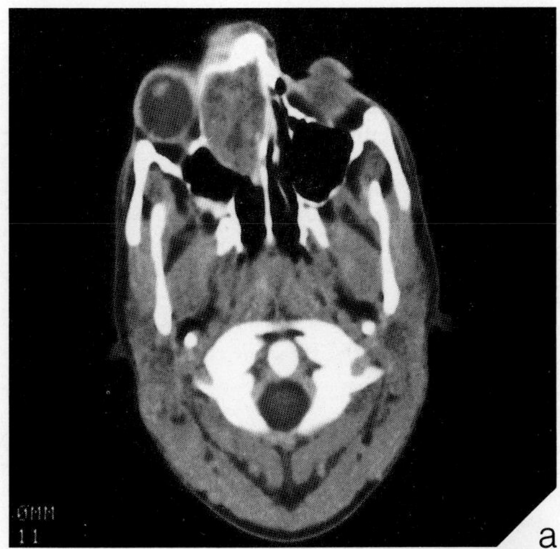

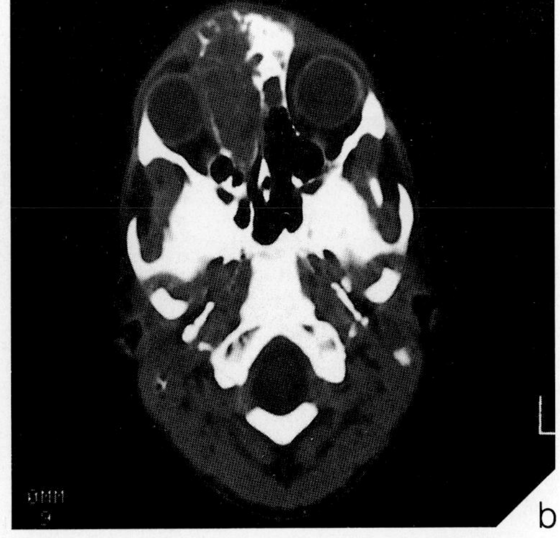

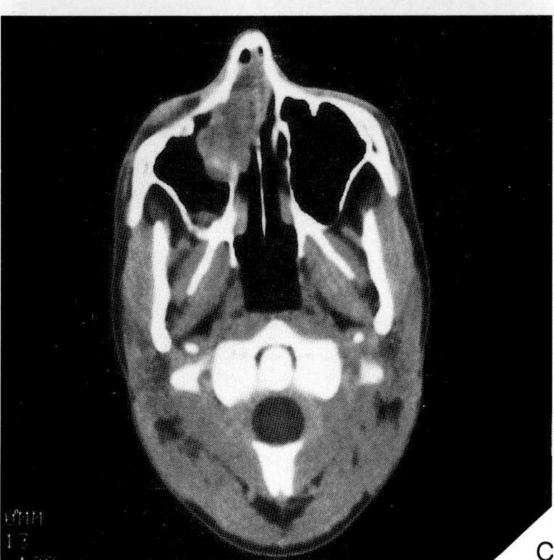

Fig. 2.18 Olfactory esthesioneuroblastoma. *This 16-year-old boy presented with nasal obstruction of recent onset. **a** An axial CT scan shows a large expansile mass in the right nasal cavity. The medial wall of the orbit is bowed outward, displacing the globe laterally. The anteromedial wall of the maxillary sinus is displaced but appears intact. **b** A more cephalic cut shows expansion of the entire ethmoid labyrinth by tumor with extensive bone destruction anteriorly. The lamina papyracea is displaced laterally and abuts the globe. A portion of the lamina papyracea has been destroyed by the tumor. **c** A cut, at the level of the maxillary sinuses (caudal to **a**), shows destruction of the ethmomaxillary angle with extension of the tumor into the maxillary sinus. (The mucosal thickening in the posterior portion of the right maxillary sinus is not part of the tumor.)*

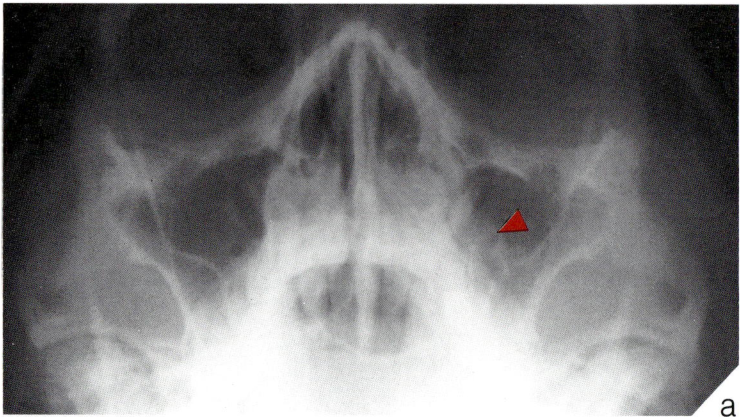

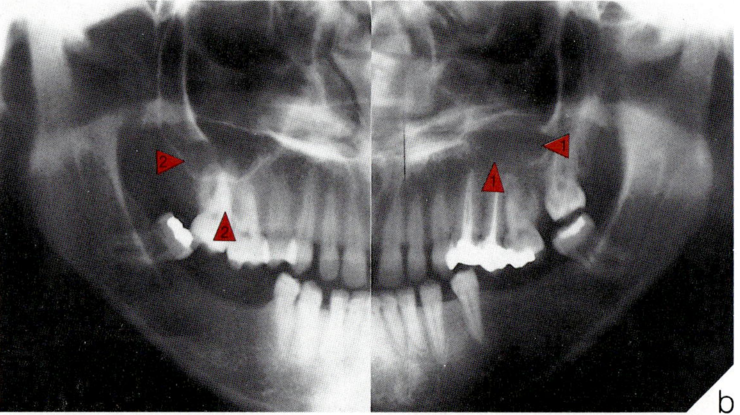

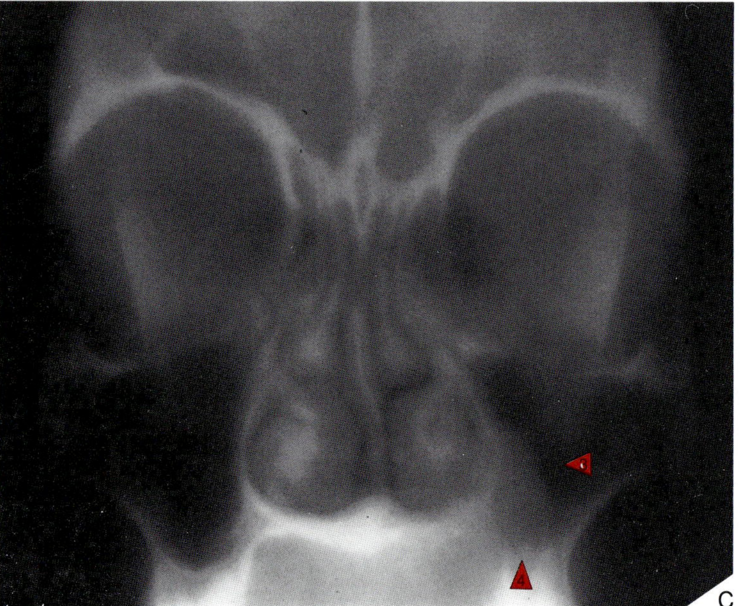

Fig. 2.19 Adenoid cystic carcinoma of the maxillary sinus. *This 26-year-old woman was believed to have an impacted wisdom tooth. A panoramic tomogram demonstrated an unexpected abnormality of the maxilla. **a** A Waters view demonstrates a soft-tissue mass (arrow) in the medial aspect of the left maxillary sinus. The rounded surface of the mass (profiled by air) suggests a benign retention cyst. **b** A panoramic tomogram shows localized bone destruction (arrows 1) in the floor of the left maxillary sinus. Compare with normal right side (arrows 2). **c** A complex-motion tomogram (coronal projection) shows the mass (arrow 3), outlined by air, in the inferomedial portion of the left maxillary sinus. There is bone destruction (arrow 4) at the junction of the alveolus with the hard palate, indicating the malignant nature of the lesion. **d** The delayed phase of an MDP bone scan (anterior view) shows increased uptake indicating an osteoblastic response. **e** An axial CT cut through the upper portion of the tumor shows its hemispheric configuration. Although this appearance might suggest a benign retention cyst, there is destruction of the medial antral wall adjacent to the mass, confirming its malignant nature. **f** A more caudal cut shows extensive destruction of the posterior wall of the maxillary sinus with extension of the tumor into the soft tissues. The medial wall of the maxillary sinus is both displaced and invaded by tumor. **g** A coronal CT cut shows focal destruction of the hard palate and nearby medial antral wall by the tumor. The relations of the soft-tissue mass as well as the bone destruction, are seen more clearly than on the complex-motion tomogram in **c.** (Reproduced with permission from Noyek, Greyson, 1985.)*

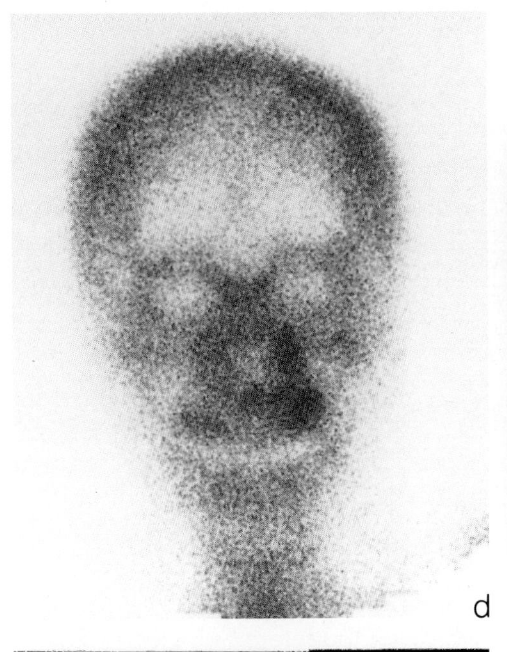

d

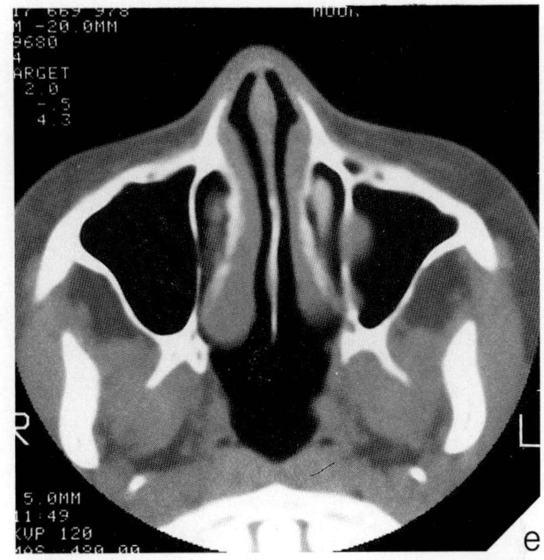

e

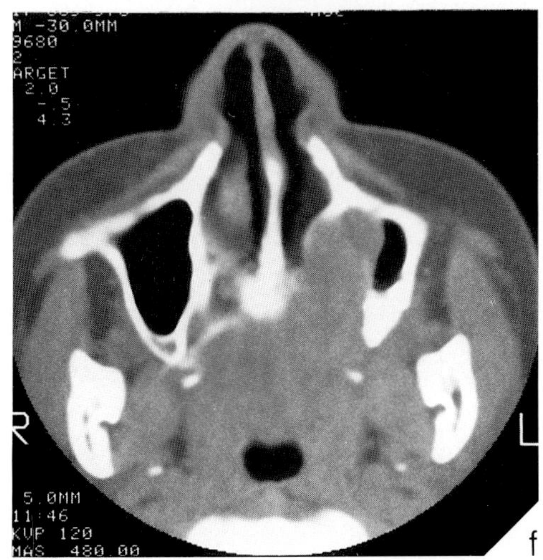

f

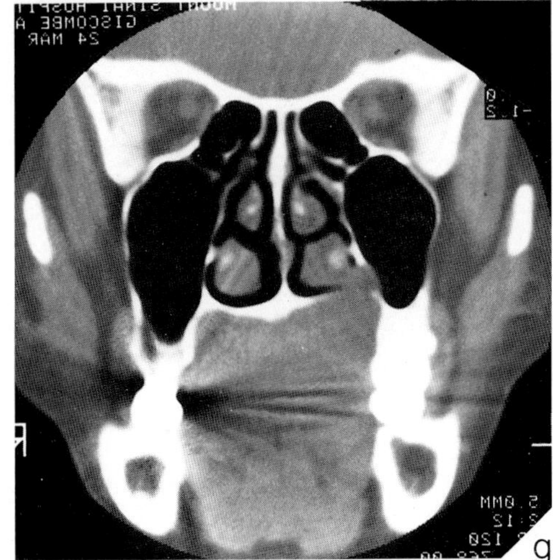

g

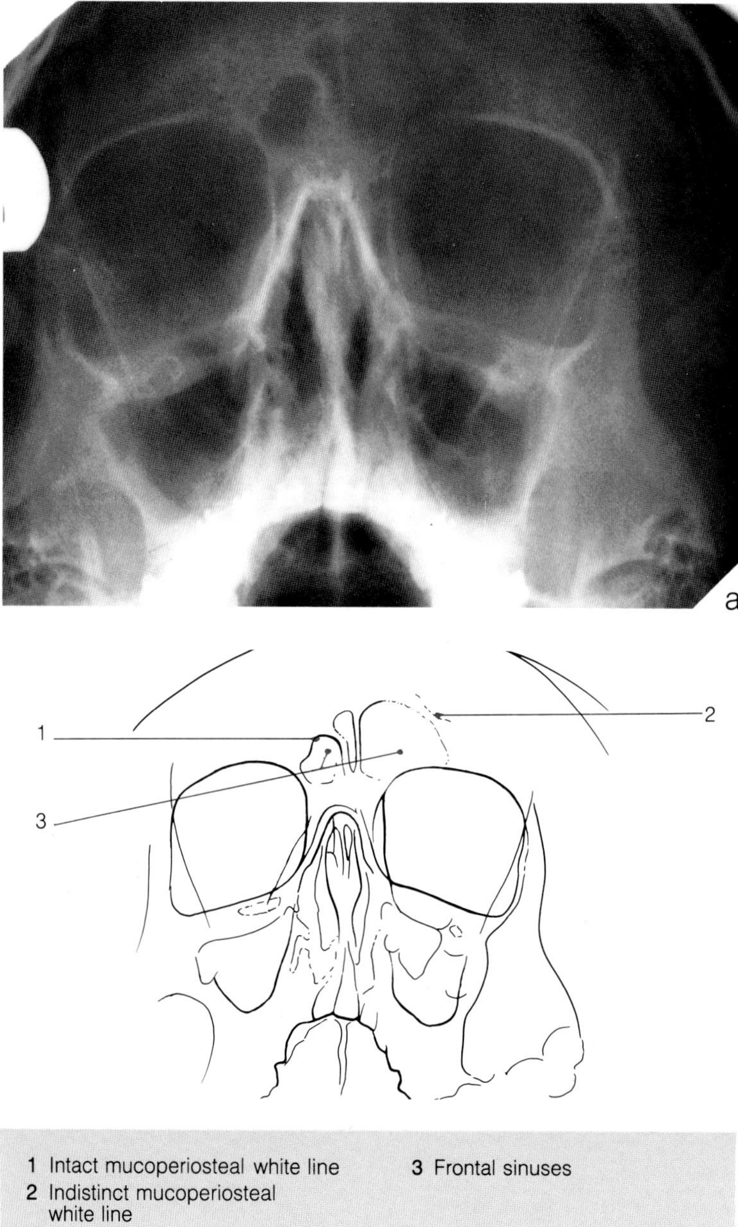

1 Intact mucoperiosteal white line   3 Frontal sinuses
2 Indistinct mucoperiosteal
  white line

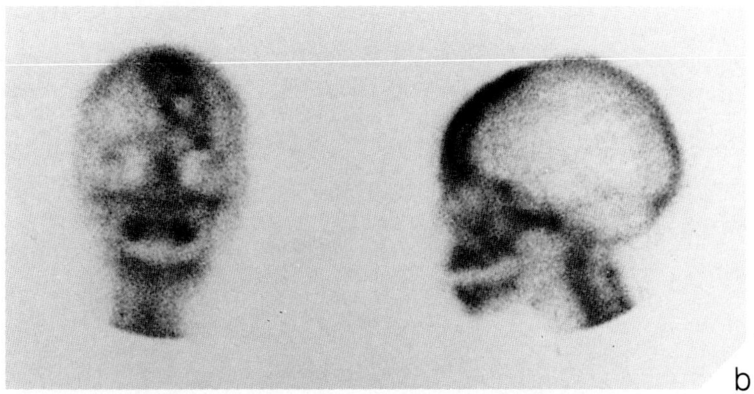

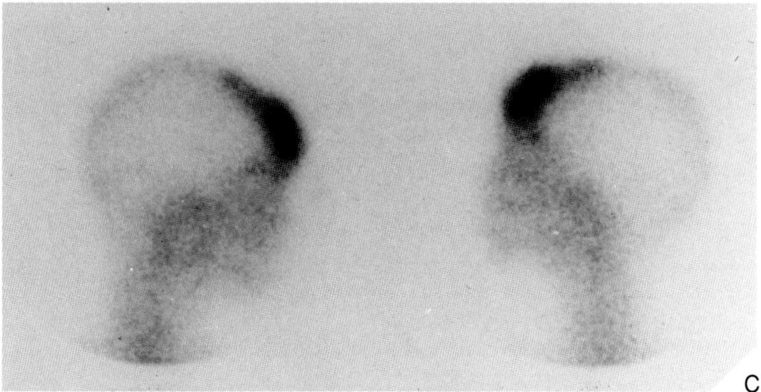

Fig. 2.20 Frontal sinusitis complicated by osteomyelitis. *This 12-year-old girl presented with symptoms of acute purulent frontal sinusitis. **a** A Waters view demonstrates clouding of left frontal sinus. There is absence of the sharp mucoperiosteal white line that normally marginates the frontal sinus, indicating that the infection has extended into the adjacent frontal bone (compare with normal right frontal sinus). **b** A Waters (left) and left lateral views of an MDP bone scan (delayed phase) show a large area of increased uptake in the frontal bone. Within the area of increased uptake there is a focus of decreased uptake which was found at operation to represent devitalized bone and early sequestrum formation. Increased uptake of MDP and other bone-seeking radionuclides reflects the osteoblastic response associated with osteomyelitis. **c** Gallium citrate scintiscans (left and right lateral views) show marked uptake of the radionuclide in the frontal bone. Gallium citrate is taken up by metabolically active leukocytes; the zone of increased uptake roughly corresponds to the inflammatory focus. (Reproduced with permission from Noyek et al, 1984.)*

Nasopharynx

The nasopharynx is difficult to evaluate clinically. A conventional mirror examination, even in skilled hands, provides limited information. While the improved optics of flexible telescopes allow the operator to assess the degree of airway obstruction and provide an excellent view of the nasopharyngeal mucosa, submucosal tumor extension cannot be detected by this means. Neither mirror nor telescope nasopharyngography can be carried out easily in an infant or child.

Because of the limitations of clinical examination, the conventional lateral radiograph remains the best means of identifying adenoidal hypertrophy (or postoperative regrowth of the adenoids) and obtaining an accurate estimate of the residual postnasal air space (see Fig. 2.20). Nasopha-ryngeal tumors (e.g., carcinoma, juvenile angiofibroma, chordoma) can extend intracranially. These tumors can also involve the cavernous sinus, orbital apex, basilar foramina, and other nearby structures. A meticulous CT or MRI examination—including images in the coronal and sagittal plane—is essential for effective treatment planning in patients with nasopharyngeal neoplasms (Figs. 3.1, 3.2).

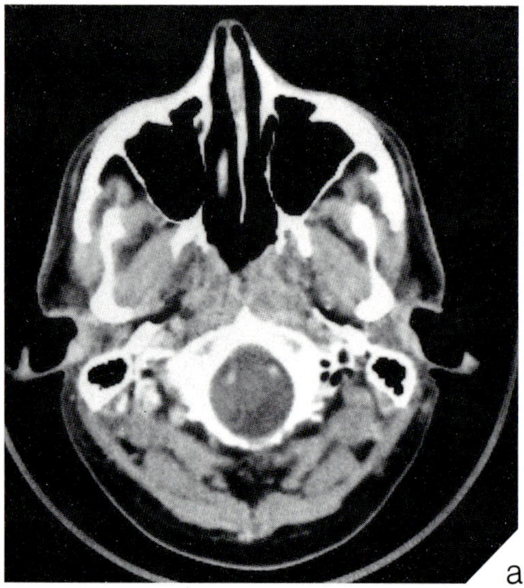
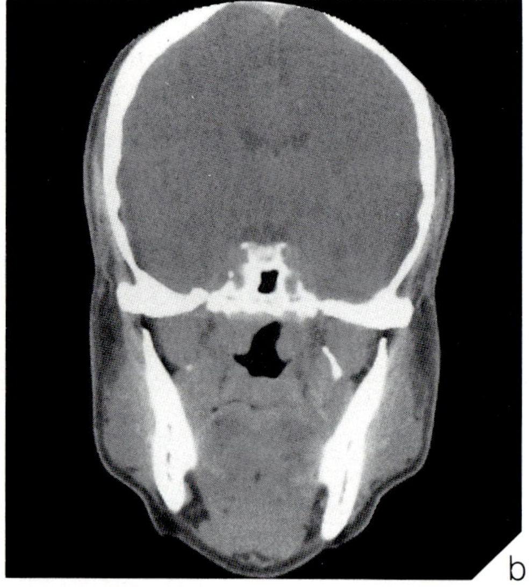

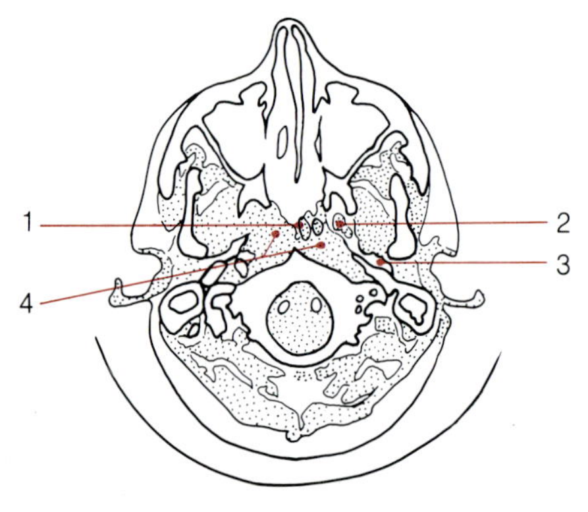

1 Tumor	4 Longus colli muscles
2 Intact fascial plane	
3 Eustachian tube	

Fig. 3.1 Small nasopharyngeal carcinoma with focal mucosal and submucosal involvement only. *This 36-year-old man presented with a single metastatic lymph node in the right deep cervical chain. **a** An axial CT scan at the level of the eustachean tubes shows a small soft-tissue mass in the left fossa of Rosenmuller region (compare with normal right side). There is no infiltration of the deep fascial planes or tensor muscles. **b** A coronal scan shows fullness of the soft tissues of the roof and right lateral aspect of the nasopharynx; compare normal right side. The fascial planes (demarcated by the surrounding fat, which is less dense) are intact.*

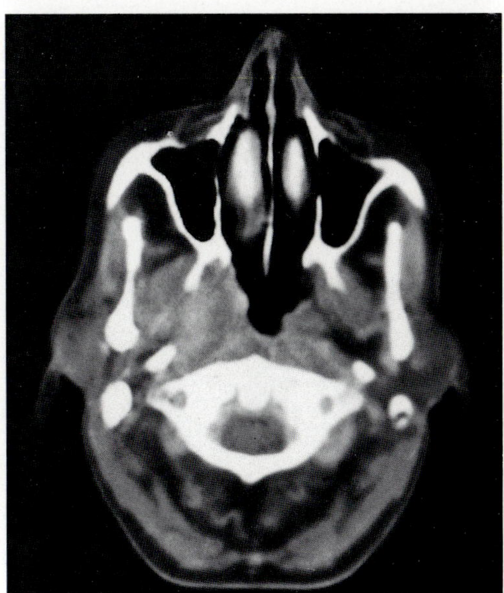

Fig. 3.2 Large, deeply infiltrating carcinoma of the nasopharynx. *This 64-year-old woman presented with a persistent serous middle-ear effusion on the right. An axial CT scan demonstrates a soft-tissue mass in the right lateral aspect of the nasopharynx in the region of the fossa of Rosenmuller. The tumor infiltrates deeply and involves the eustachian tube. Note that the fascial planes have been destroyed by the advancing neoplasm (compare normal left side).*

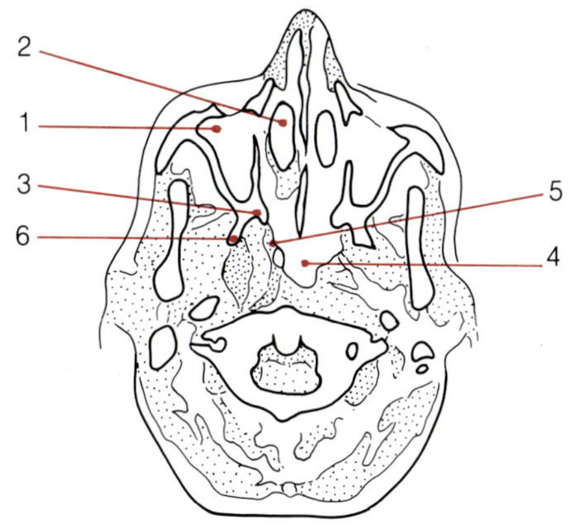

1 Maxillary sinus
2 Inferior turbinate
3 Right medial
  pterygoid plate
4 Nasopharyngeal
  air space
5 Tumor
6 Right lateral
  pterygoid plate

Orbital Extension of Diseases of the Nasal Cavity and Paranasal Sinuses

Orbital extension is a significant complication of infections, mucoceles, and neoplasms of the nasal cavity and paranasal sinuses, and has important therapeutic implications. While plain films and complex-motion tomography often provide useful information (Fig. 4.1), only CT or MRI can document the true extent of orbital involvement (Figs. 4.2–4.4). CT also plays an important role in the management of major cranioorbitofacial injuries (see Chapter 7 on maxillofacial skeleton).

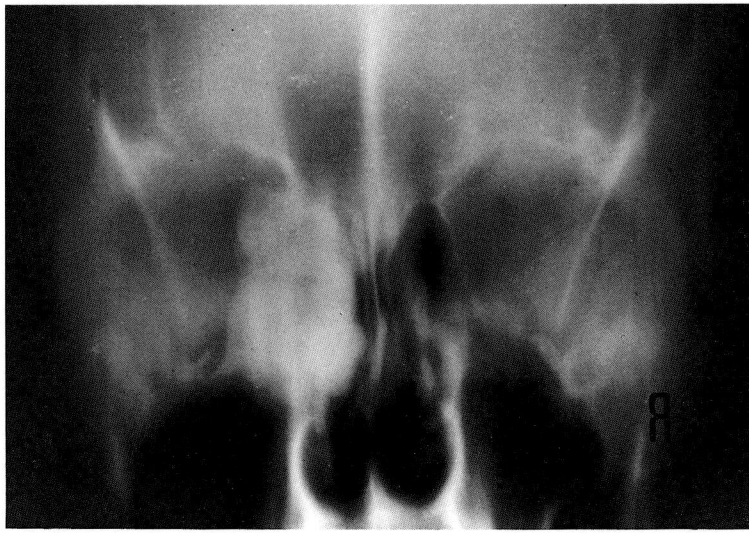

Fig. 4.1 Ethmoid osteoma with orbital extension. *A coronal complex-motion tomogram shows a lobulated osteoma arising in the ethmoid labyrinth. The bony mass encroaches on the nasal cavity and the superomedial angle of the maxillary sinus and extends into the orbit causing proptosis. Although the tumor is benign, it has eroded and destroyed the lamina papyracea (compare intact lamina papyracea on opposite side). (Reproduced with permission from Noyek et al, 1987.)*

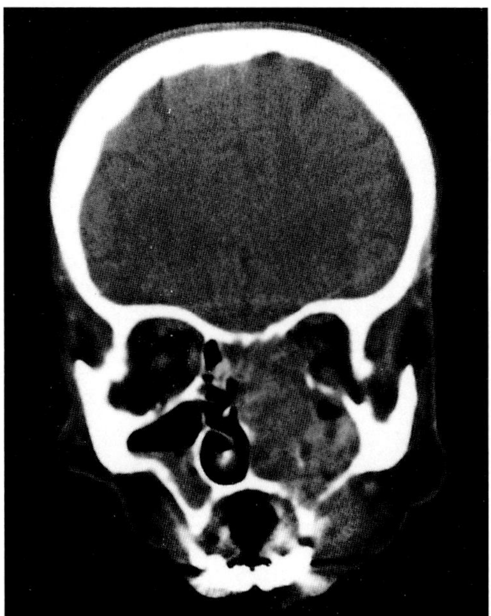

Fig. 4.2 Carcinoma of the maxillary sinus with orbital invasion. *A coronal CT scan shows intraorbital extension from a large carcinoma arising in the right maxillary sinus. The tumor extends medially into the nasal cavity, superiorly into the ethmoid labyrinth; and anterolaterally into the oral cavity. There is obvious extension of tumor into the orbit with destruction of the normal bony landmarks; the floor of the orbit (roof of the maxillary sinus) is fragmented (compare with normal bony structures of left orbit.) In this plane the bony floor of the anterior cranial fossa appears intact. A fluid level is present in the left maxillary sinus.*

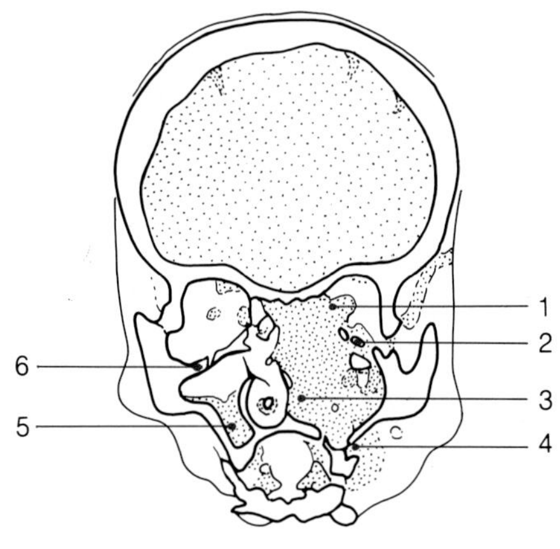

1 Extension into orbit	**4** Bone destruction
2 Fragmented floor of orbit	**5** Fluid in maxillary sinus
3 Tumor	**6** Normal orbit floor

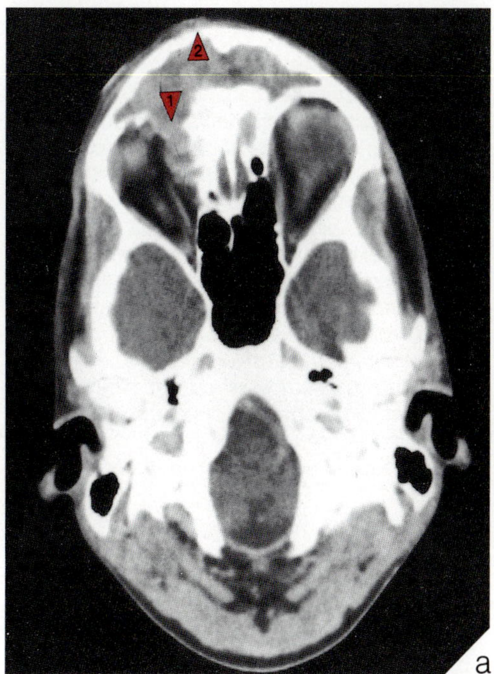 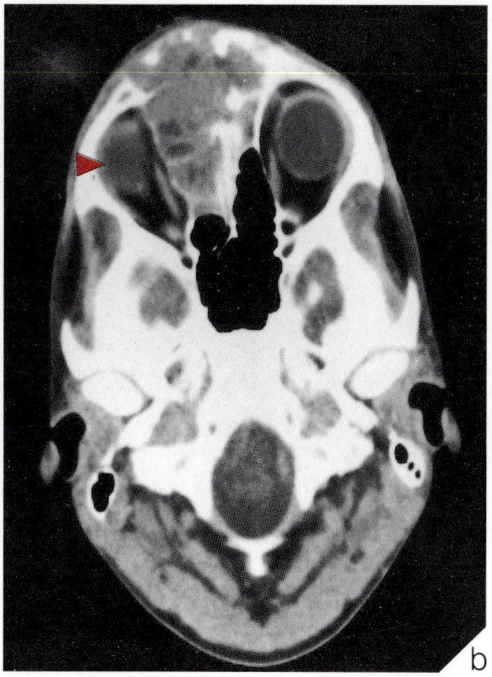

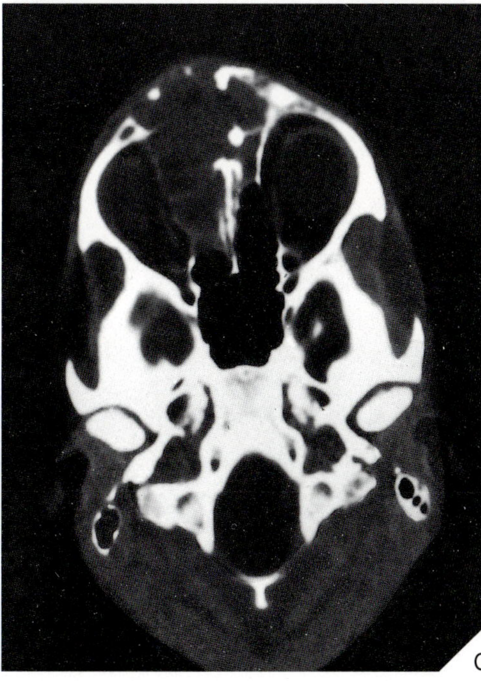

Fig. 4.3 Olfactory esthesioneuroblastoma with orbital extension. *a Axial CT cuts of the same patient shown in Fig. 2.18. The tumor, which originated in the nasal cavity, has extended into both frontal sinuses, and posterolaterally into the right ethmoid labyrinth and orbit. There is focal bone destruction at the superomedial angle of the right orbit (arrow 1). Thickening of soft tissues anterior to the right frontal sinus is tumor (arrow 2). b A more caudal cut (5 mm below a) shows extensive destruction of the anterior wall of the frontal sinus. On this cut, the lamina papyracea is demineralized and displaced into the right orbit, displacing the globe (arrow) laterally. c A bone window of the same cut better shows the bone destruction in the anterior wall of the frontal sinus and superomedial wall of the right orbit. A thorough CT examination (which sometimes entails multiple scanning planes and reconstructions, as well as soft-tissue and bone windows) is essential for planning surgery and/or radiation therapy in patients with malignant tumors of the paranasal sinuses and nasal cavity.*

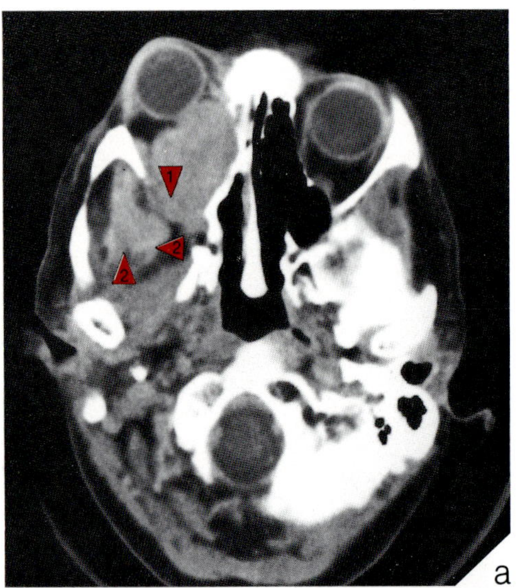

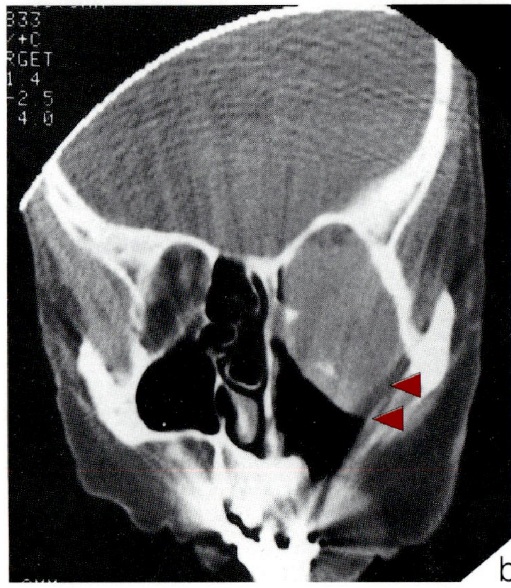

Fig. 4.4 Carcinoma of the maxillary sinus with orbital invasion. *This 65-year-old woman had previously undergone a partial maxillectomy for an acinic cell carcinoma of the right maxillary sinus and returned 2 years later with diplopia and recurrence of pain. **a** An axial CT cut demonstrates a huge lobulated tumor in the right orbit, which displaces the globe anteriorly. There is extensive bone destruction (arrow 1) of the lateral wall of the orbit. However, the structures of the infratemporal fossa (arrows 2) are normal. **b** On the coronal scan the tumor fills the orbit. There is extensive destruction of the floor of the orbit and tumor bulges inferiorly into the maxillary sinus, where it is sharply profiled by air. Note absence of anterolateral wall of the maxillary sinus (arrows), which was resected during the previous operation.*

Skull Base

The skull base—the bony terrain between the facial skeleton and related structures below and the three cranial fossae and their contents above—could not be evaluated accurately before the advent of contemporary imaging techniques. The evolution of skull-base surgery has been dependent on, and nurtured by, the radiologist's ability to localize precisely and to delineate pathology from the cribriform plate to the foramen magnum. The foramina, which transmit neurovascular structures and serve as a pathway between the cranial contents and the visceral spaces below the skull base, can now be explored radiologically.

Careful radiologic evaluation of the skull base is essential in patients with malignant tumors of the paranasal sinuses and nasopharynx, as well those with benign lesions that tend to extend intracranially such as juvenile angiofibromas and chordomas. Close collaboration between the clinician and radiologist is the key to success in imaging this complex region.

Plain films and complex-motion tomograms are often very informative in patients with lesions of the skull base (Fig. 5.1). The submentovertical ("base") projection is particularly useful for evaluating the foramina (Fig. 5.2). Complex-motion tomograms accurately depict bone destruction in the frontal and sagittal planes (Fig. 5.3). However, CT detects soft-tissue pathology as well and is the preferred examination, especially for lesions involving the foramina (Figs. 5.4, 5.5). (Sagittal tomograms show bone detail more clearly than sagittal CT reformations, and may help in some cases.)

To ensure the maximum diagnostic yield, the CT examination must be carefully planned and closely monitored. Subtle pathologic changes can often be detected by tailoring the technical aspects of the examination to the individual patient and to the specific clinical problem.

MRI promises to be an important new tool for evaluating this complex anatomic region. MRI depicts the soft tissues of the skull base vividly not only in the axial and coronal planes, but in the all-important sagittal plane. By increasing the T2-relaxation time, the cerebrospinal fluid pathways can be visualized without contrast injection, eliminating the need for myelography in patients with suspected lesions in the vicinity of the clivus and foramen magnum.

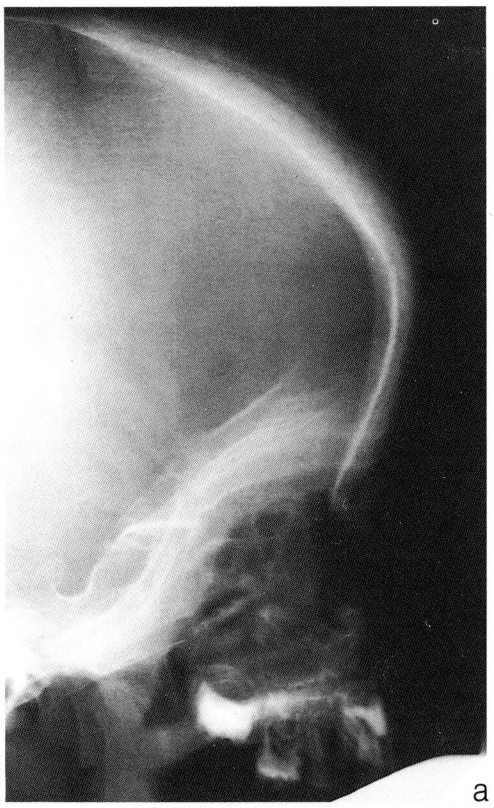

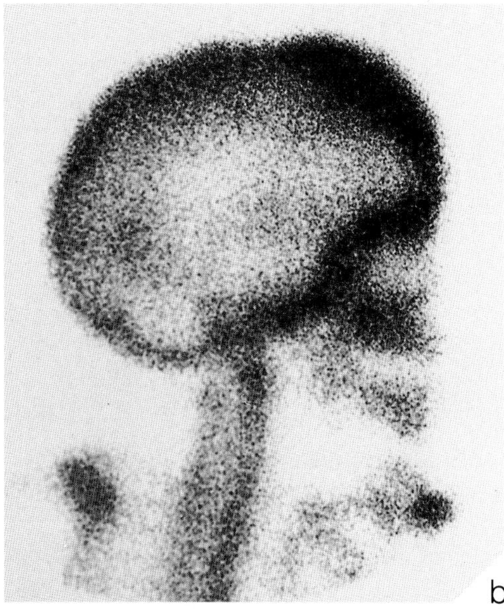

Fig. 5.1 Fibrous dysplasla. *a Lateral skull film of a 2-year-old boy shows bone thickening and sclerosis involving the frontal bone and the floor of the anterior cranial fossa.* ***b*** *The delayed phase of a radionuclide bone scan (right lateral view) confirms the osteoblastic nature of the lesion.*

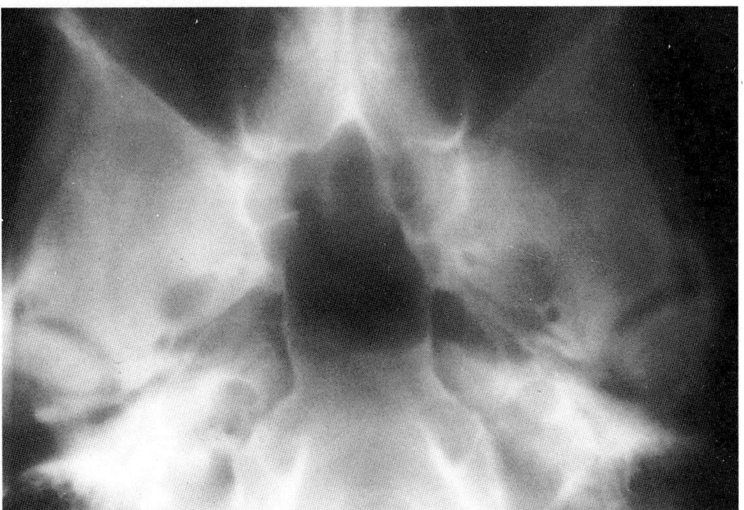

Fig. 5.2 Expansion of foramen ovale by malignant schwannoma.
Base view of the skull shows markedly expanded left foramen ovale, with indistinct margins; compare normal right foramen ovale. The margins are indistinct. The foramen spinosum is not involved.

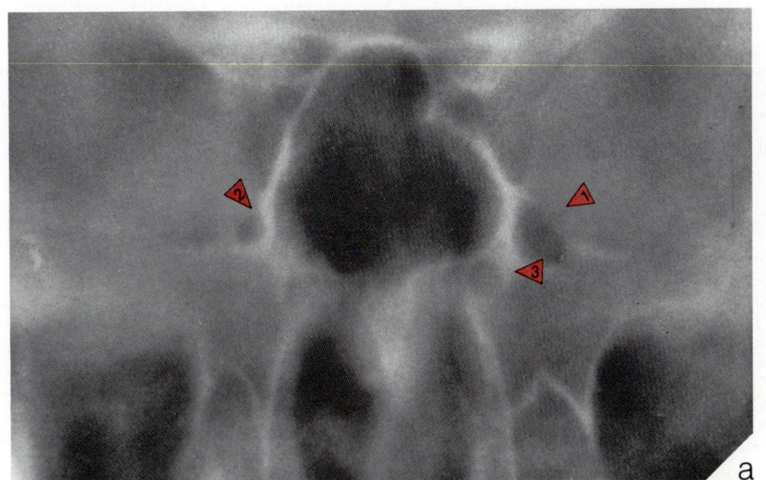

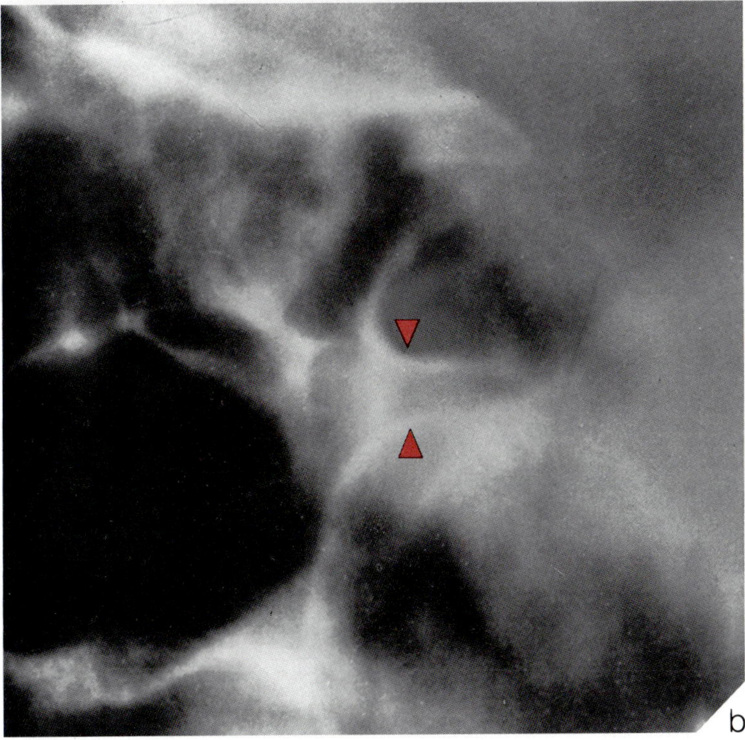

Fig. 5.3 Neurofibroma enlarging the foramen rotundum. *a Coronal complex-motion tomogram demonstrates enlargement of the left foramen rotundum (arrow 1) by a neurofibroma of the maxillary nerve in a patient with neurofibromatosis (von Recklinghausen's disease). Compare normal foramen rotundum on the right (arrow 2). The vidian canal in the floor of the left sphenoid sinus is indicated (arrow 3). b Sagittal tomogram shows expansion of the bony canal by the tumor (arrows). (Reproduced with permission from Noyek et al, 1982.)*

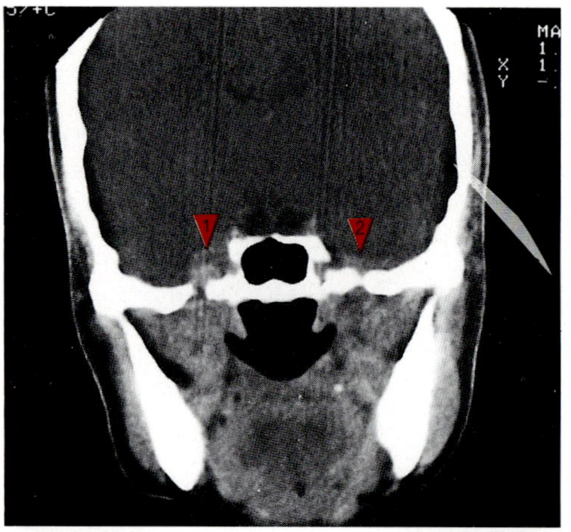

Fig. 5.4 Malignant schwannoma of the trigeminal nerve. *This 40-year-old woman presented with numbness in the distribution of the third division of the trigeminal nerve on the left. A coronal CT scan demonstrates a small enhancing tumor mass (arrow 1) projecting from foramen ovale into the left middle cranial fossa. The normal right foramen ovale is indicated (arrow 2). The paired cartilaginous eustachian tubal cushions are seen as conical structures projecting into the nasopharyngeal air column. (Reproduced with permission from Noyek et al, 1982.)*

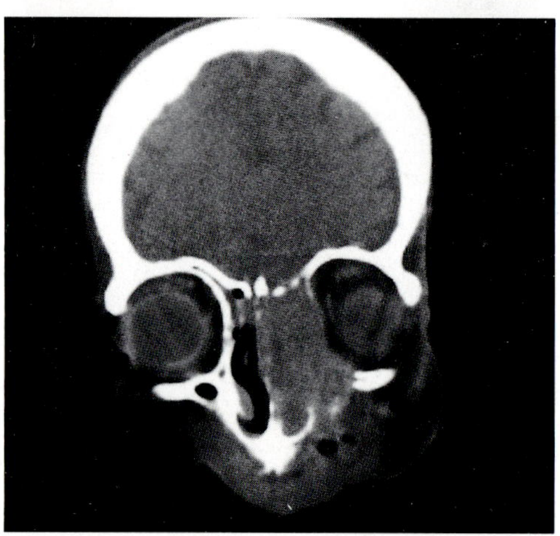

Fig. 5.5 Maxillary sinus carcinoma with intracranial extension. *Coronal CT scan of the same patient as shown in Fig. 4.2. The left maxillary sinus is filled with tumor, which has extended beyond the confines of the sinus into the nasal cavity and ethmoid labyrinth and inferolaterally into the deep facial soft tissues. Cephalic extension of the tumor has disrupted the floor of the anterior cranial fossa. The tumor has also invaded the orbit.*

*I*ntracranial Relationships of Otorhinologic Disorders

CT has revolutionized the diagnosis and management of intracranial disease. Its major role for the otolaryngologist, in this regard, has been its ability to demonstrate intracranial extension of disease processes arising in the paranasal sinuses (Figs. 6.1, 6.2) or the middle-ear cleft. Although an upright film may sometimes demonstrate a gas–fluid level in an intracranial abscess secondary to sinusitis or mastoiditis, most intracranial complications of otolaryngologic disease cannot be detected by conventional radiographic techniques.

CT can also characterize intracranial disorders that encroach on the terrain of the otolaryngologist. A meningocele or meningoencephalocele, for example, can present as a unilateral mass in the nasal cavity (Figs. 6.3, 6.4). Intracranial neoplasms may extend into the frontal sinus, ethmoid labyrinth, or orbit (Fig. 6.5). By combining CT with intrathecal administration of a low osmolality nonionic contrast agent (e.g., iohexal or iopamidol), active cerebrospinal fluid leaks can be identified and accurately localized (Fig. 6.6).

While its precise role remains to be defined, MRI is likely to supplant CT as the diagnostic modality of choice in the investigation of these complex problems.

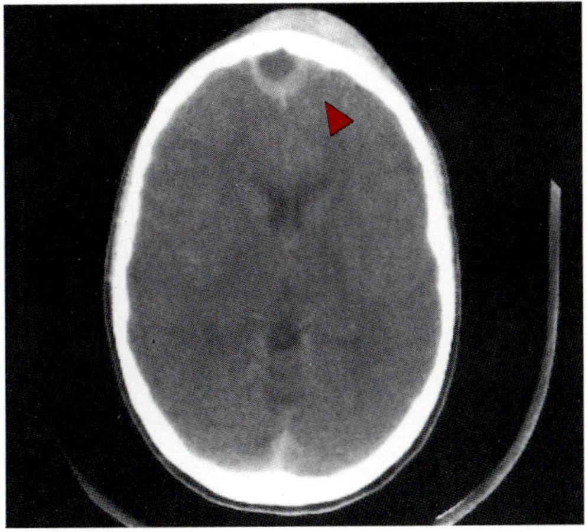

Fig. 6.1 Extradural abscess, osteomyelitis, and Pott's puffy tumor secondary to frontal sinusitis. *Same patient as shown in Fig. 2.20. A contrast-enhanced axial CT scan shows a midline extraaxial mass with an enhancing rim (arrow), which represents an extradural abscess secondary to extension of the infection through the inner table. Also note soft-tissue swelling over the frontal bone due to extension of the pyogenic infection through the outer table (Pott's puffy tumor). (Reproduced with permission from Noyek et al, 1984.)*

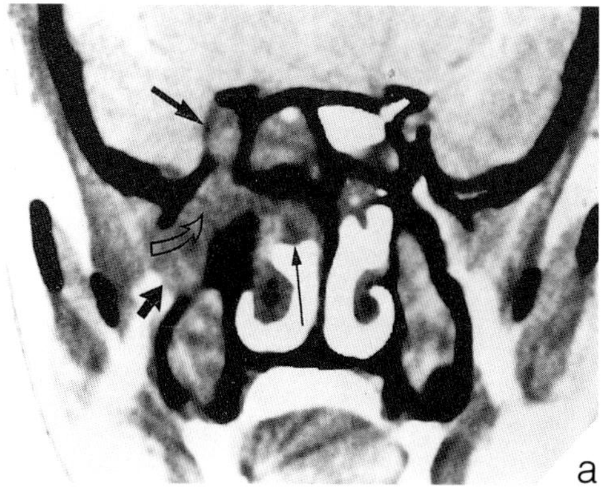

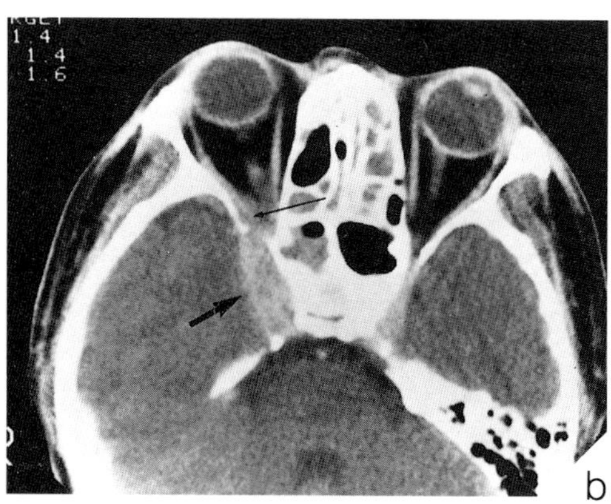

a

b

Fig. 6.2 Carcinoma of the nasopharynx with intracranial extension. *a Coronal CT shows extension of the tumor into the middle cranial fossa* (medium arrow) *and inferiorly through the inferior orbital fissure* (short, solid arrow) *which is markedly widened* (open arrow). *Tumor is also present in the superior aspect of the nasal cavity* (thin arrow). *There is soft-tissue thicken-* ing within the sphenoid sinus; although CT cannot differentiate between tumor and infection, the latter would certainly be suspect. *b The axial projection shows tumor at the apex of the right orbit* (thin arrow) *which extends as an enhancing mass into the right cavernous sinus* (thick arrow). *(Courtesy of E.E. Kassel.)*

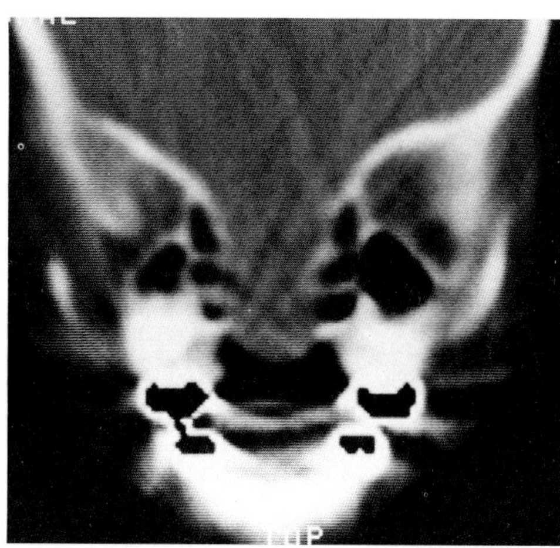

Fig. 6.3 Sphenoid encephalocele in an infant. *A coronal CT scan shows a huge encephalocele herniating into the ethmoid labyrinth through a bony defect in the floor of the anterior cranial fossa. (Reproduced with permission from Fitz, Noyek, 1981.)*

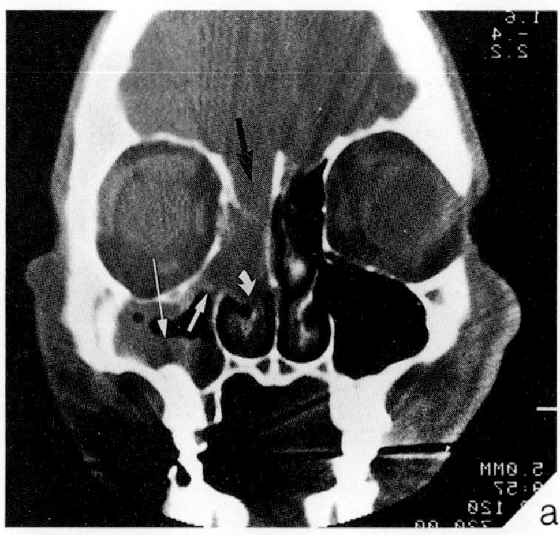

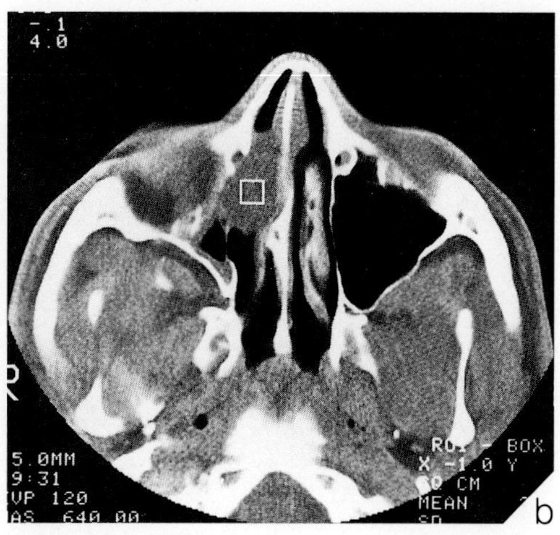

Fig. 6.4 Ethmoid encephalocele in an adult. *This man presented with a stuffy nose and sinusitis. Physical examination revealed a fleshy nasal polyp. **a** A coronal CT scan demonstrates the unilateral herniation of an encephalocele through the roof of the ethmoid labyrinth (cribriform plate) on the right (black arrow). The lower margin of the encephalocele encroaches on the nasal cavity (curved arrow). The mass also obstructs the meatus of the ipsi-* *lateral maxillary sinus (medium white arrow) (note fluid level; thin arrow). **b** The axial scan shows a polypoid mass within the right nasal cavity. CT number is 23 Hounsfield units, consistent with brain tissue. (Note: Forewarned by the CT scan that this patient's nasal "polyp" was of intracranial origin, the otolaryngologist was able to avoid an inappropriate—and potentially catastrophic—intranasal procedure.)*

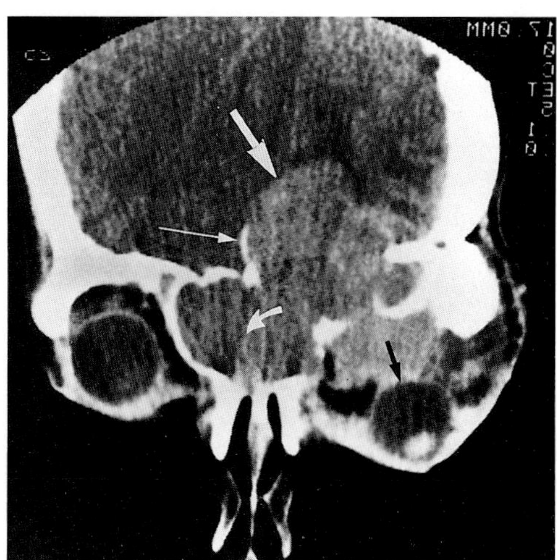

Fig. 6.5 Subfrontal meningioma in the orbit and frontal sinuses. *A coronal CT shows a large subfrontal meningioma, invading the left orbit and both frontal sinuses (curved arrow), extending intracranially (medium white arrow). There is extensive destruction and fragmentation of the floor of the anterior cranial fossa on the left. A bone fragment is displaced across the midline (thin arrow). The tumor extends through the roof of the orbit, displacing the globe (black arrow) inferiorly and laterally. (Courtesy of E.E. Kassel.)*

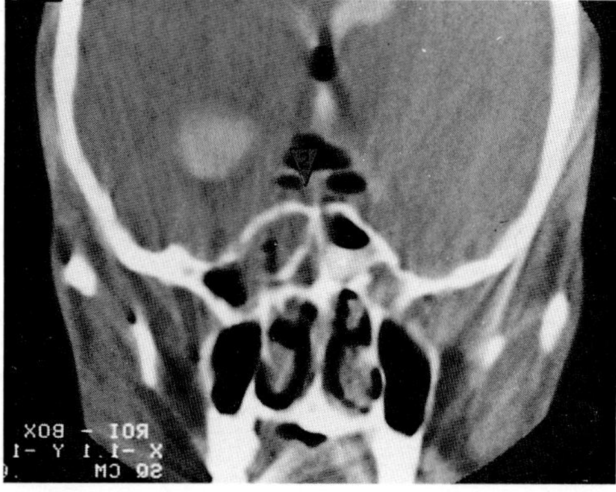

Fig. 6.6 Cerebrospinal fluid leak due to fracture of sphenoid sinus. *CSF rhinorrhea following a basal skull fracture. A coronal CT scan after intrathecal injection of metrizamide shows contrast material in the left sphenoid sinus; the CSF fistula is at a sinus roof fracture (arrow 2).*

Maxillofacial Skeleton

Congenital malformations of the maxillofacial skeleton may occur in isolation or as part of a syndrome. Although a great deal can often be learned from conventional radiographs and complex-motion tomography, CT is often needed for complete assessment of distorted anatomic relations (Fig. 7.1). With meticulous technique, bony and soft-tissue abnormalities can be precisely deline-ated even in infants and young children. MRI promises to be very useful in patients with associated skull base defects or herniation of intracranial contents.

A careful radiologic assessment is an integral part of the management of maxillofacial trauma. Plain films usually suffice in patients with isolated fractures of the nasal bones and zygoma (Fig. 7.2). Complex-motion tomograms provide important additional information in patients with orbital-floor fractures (Fig. 7.3). CT plays an important role in the management of complex maxillofacial injuries, both to document the extent of the fractures and to exclude associated injuries of the intracranial contents and the orbital soft tissues (e.g., disruption of the optic nerve, dislocated lens) (Fig. 7.4).

In an acutely injured patient, the CT examination is usually limited to scanning in the axial plane. Contiguous thin slices (5 mm or less) should be obtained, as coronal and/or sagittal reconstructions (reformations) may be necessary to fully evaluate some complex fractures. A direct coronal scan is more informative than a reformatted coronal image, and can be obtained if the patient's condition permits and there is no associated cervical spine injury.

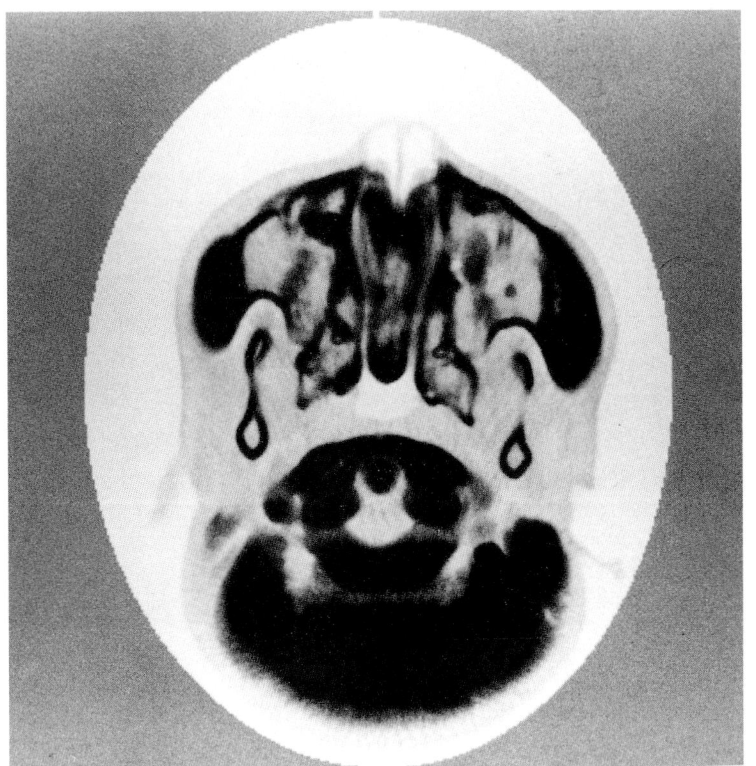

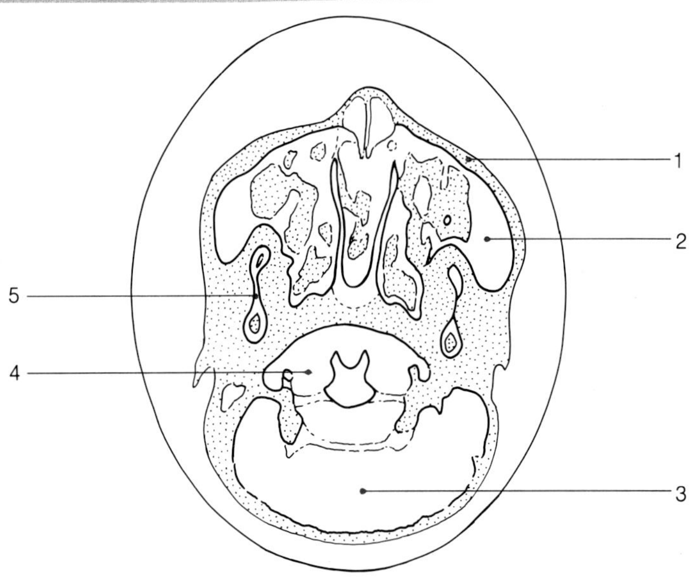

Fig. 7.1 Craniometaphyseal dysplasia. *An axial CT scan (bones appear black in this reversed image) in a child with craniometaphyseal dysplasia shows marked bony thickening of the calvarium, facial bones, mandible, and cervical spine. Progressive narrowing of cranial foramina is a characteristic feature of this rare skeletal dysplasia. CT can detect narrowing of the optic or auditory canal before irreversible nerve damage occurs. (Reproduced with permission from Fitz, Noyek, 1981.)*

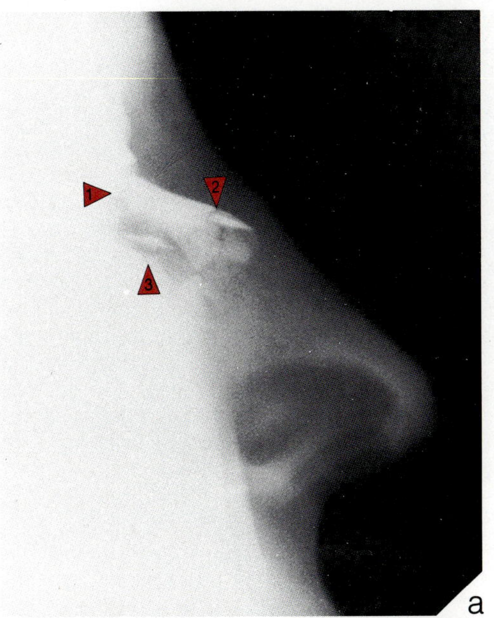

Fig. 7.2 Nasal fracture. *a* The lateral radiograph shows a fracture through the nasal process of the frontal bone with posterior displacement of the entire nasal complex (arrow 1). There is a fracture line through the distal third of the nasal bones (arrow 2) *as well. A large fracture fragment (arrow 3)* is seen just beneath the displaced nasal complex; the direction of displacement cannot be judged on this projection. *b* The Waters view shows that the arch of the nasal bones is disrupted at at least two points (arrows 4). A large, medially displaced bone fragment (arrow 5), *which corresponds to depressed fragment seen on the lateral projection, lies just below the gap in the arch on the left. (Reproduced with permission from Noyek et al, 1983.)*

a

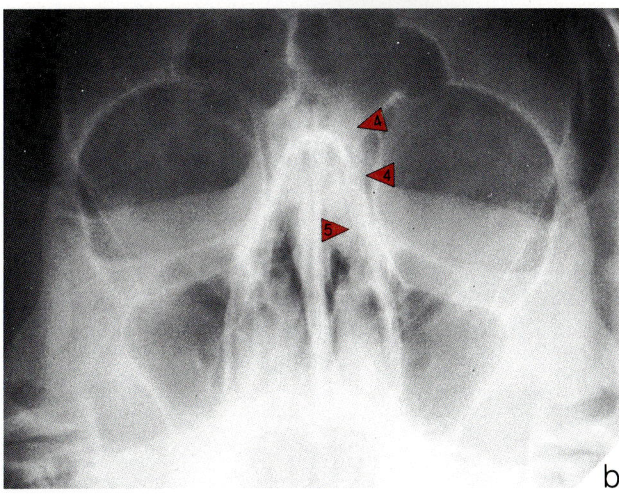

b

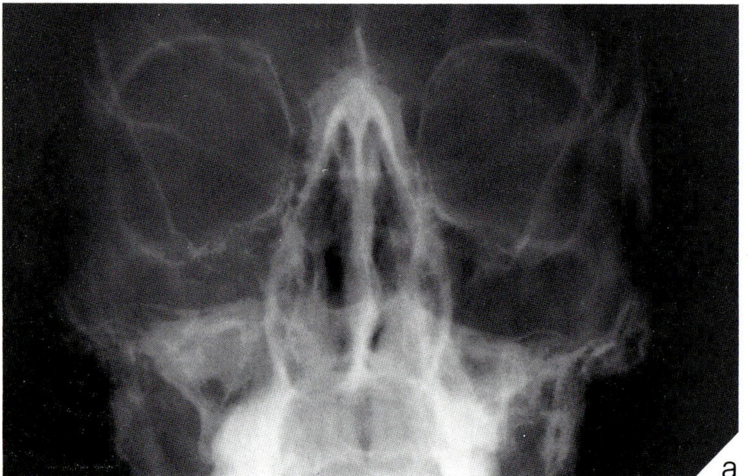

Fig. 7.3 Fracture of the orbital floor and zygoma. *a* A modified anteroposterior projection shows a fracture of the right zygoma with separation of the zygomatico-frontal suture. The lateral wall of the right orbit is displaced medially and the floor of the orbit is shattered (compare with normal structures on left.) The right maxillary sinus is opacified by blood. *b* A coronal complex-motion tomogram demonstrates the opacified right maxillary sinus and disruption of the orbital floor. A large bone fragment (arrow 5) is displaced into the right maxillary sinus.

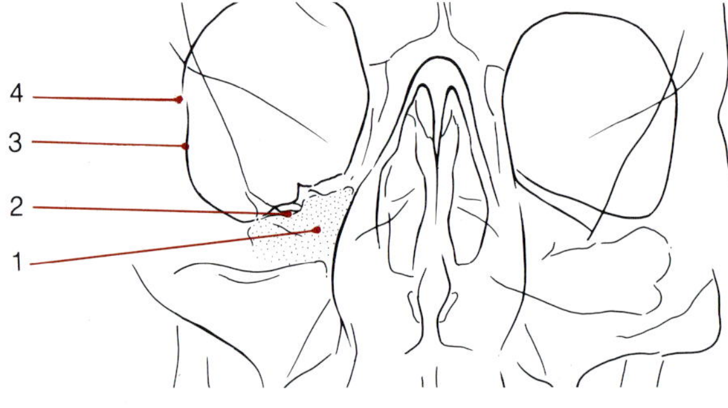

1 Opacified maxillary sinus	**4** Separation of zygomaticofrontal suture
2 Shattered floor of right orbit	**5** Bone fragment
3 Medially displaced lateral wall of orbit	

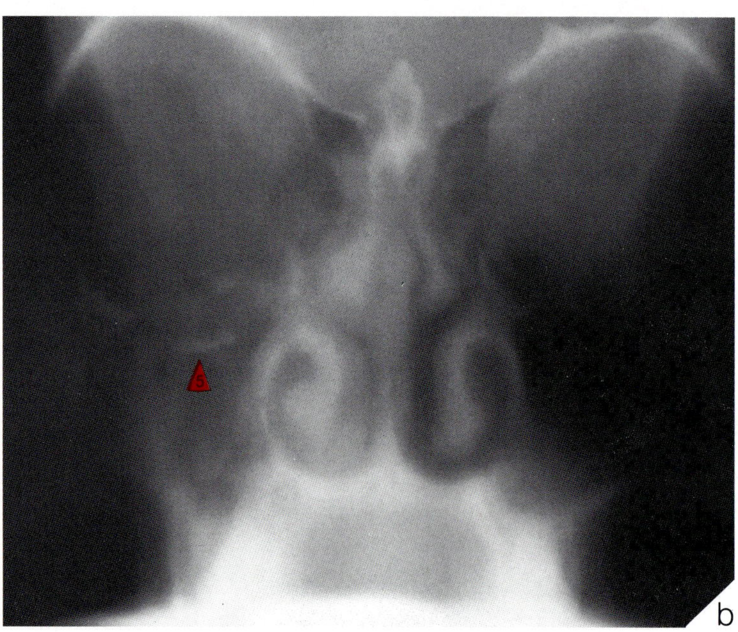

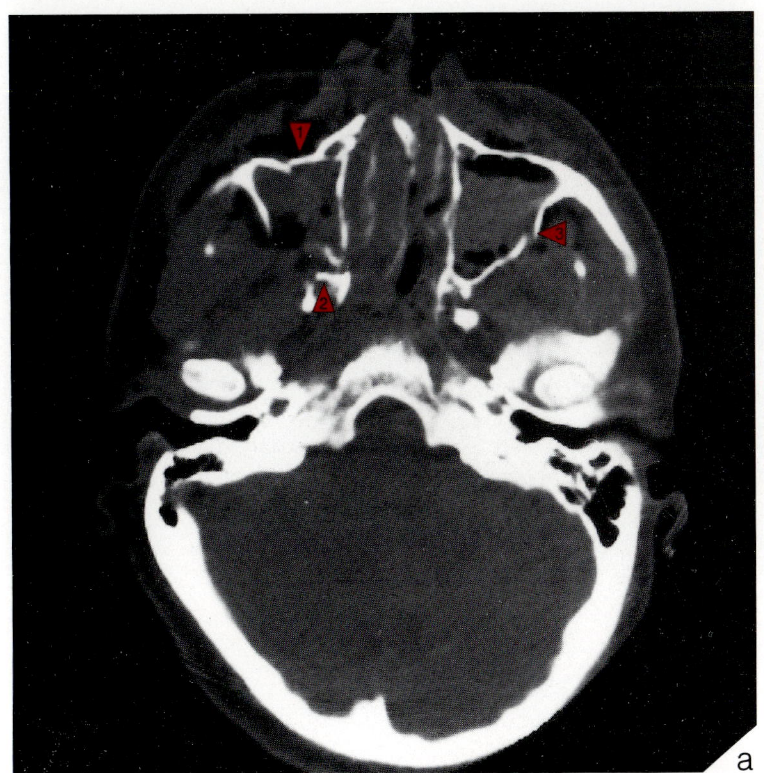

Fig. 7.4 Le Fort II fracture of the facial bones. *a* *An axial CT scan at the level of the maxillary antra demonstrates multiple fracture lines. The anterior wall of the right maxillary sinus is shattered (arrow 1); the posterior wall is disrupted; and the pterygoid plates are fractured (arrow 2). The right maxillary sinus is opacified by hemorrhage. On the left, the posterolateral wall of the maxillary sinus is fractured (arrow 3), an air–blood level is present in the sinus. Both nasal cavities are filled with blood and the lateral walls of the nasal cavities are fractured.* ***b*** *An axial CT cut at the level of the ethmoid labyrinth demonstrates total disruption of the ethmoid cells bilaterally. The left globe (arrow) is displaced laterally.*

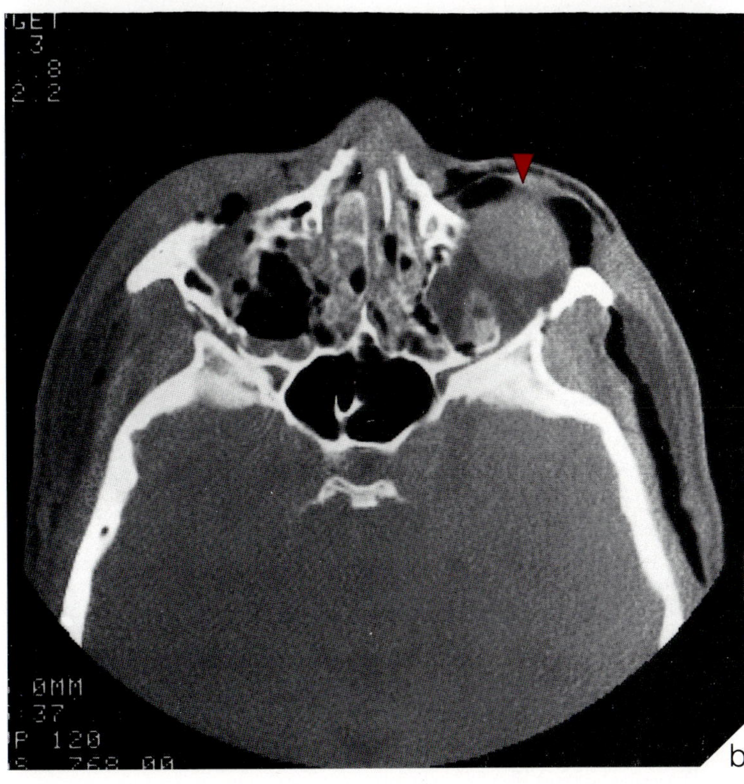

Temporomandibular Joints and Mandible

Many abnormalities of the temporomandibular (TM) joints can be assessed with plain films. Additional imaging techniques (e.g., linear, panoramic, or complex-motion tomography; radiopharmaceutical scintigraphy; CT; arthrography; MRI) may be needed to clarify a complex problem (Fig. 8.1). The radiopharmaceutical bone scan is a useful screening technique in patients with suspected inflammatory or neoplastic involvement of the TM joints; abnormal uptake warrants further investigation by thin-section tomography or CT.

Primary osteoarthritis, rheumatoid arthritis, pyrophosphate deposition disease (pseudogout), and other primary arthropathies of the TM joints, as well as degenerative osteoarthritis due to direct or surgical trauma or long-standing occlusal derangement, can be detected and followed by various imaging techniques (Fig. 8.2).

Mandibular involvement can occur in neoplastic and inflammatory diseases of the oral and perioral soft tissues. Before initiating treatment in patients with squamous cell carcinoma of the oral cavity, it is important to detect subclinical mandibular invasion. Similarly, in patients with clinical evidence of mandibular involvement, the extent of bone invasion must be documented. Extensive bone destruction is readily appreciated on conventional radiographs (Fig. 8.3), whereas focal mandibular involvement is better appreciated on periapical dental films. Panoramic tomography provides an overall view of the entire mandible (Fig. 8.4). Although panoramic tomograms demonstrate the external surface of the mandible to advantage, the inner cortical margin may not be clearly seen. Complex-motion tomography and CT allow a more detailed assessment of bone involvement. However, CT demonstrates both soft-tissue and bone pathology, and should be used for morphologic staging of advanced carcinoma of the oral cavity.

The radionuclide bone scan correlates more closely with the pathologic findings than either complex-motion tomography or CT, both of which tend to "underestimate" bone involvement. Thus the bone scan allows recognition of bone invasion in its earliest stages, before radiographic changes are apparent (Fig. 8.5). In patients with clinical mandibular involvement, the changes seen on the bone scan are invariably more extensive than those seen on conventional radiographic images or CT, and indicate the actual extent of bone disease (see Figs. 8.3b, 8.4b).

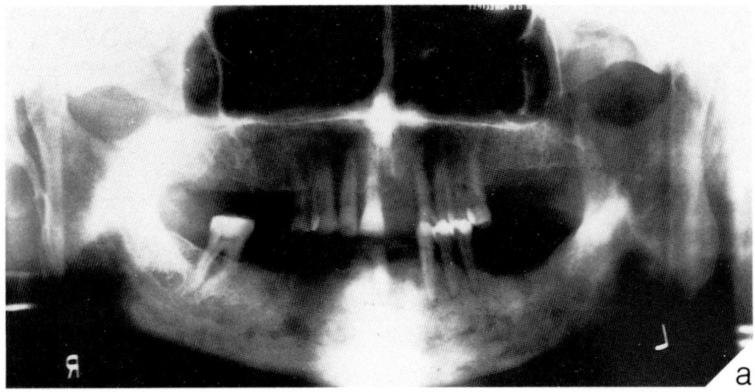

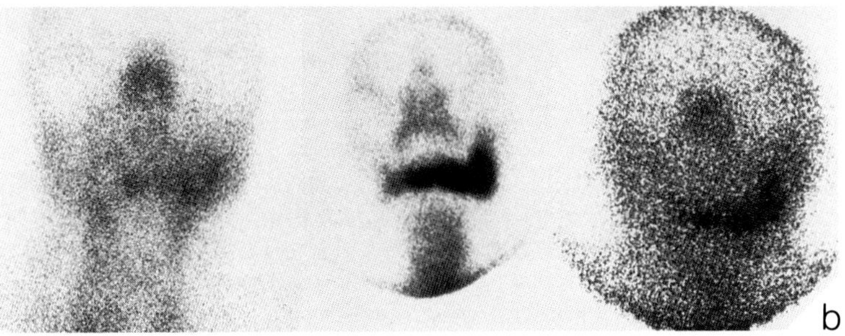

Fig. 8.1 Chronic osteomyelitis of the mandible. *The patient is a 67-year-old man with long-standing osteomyelitis of dental origin that has been refractory to treatment.* ***a*** *A panoramic tomogram shows patchy destructive changes and sclerosis of both mandibular rami and irregular thickening of the deformed alveolar ridge.* ***b*** *A composite figure shows anterior views of an MDP bone scan* (left and center) *and a subsequent gallium scan* (right). *The blood-pool phase of the bone scan* (left) *shows increased uptake, more marked on the left side, reflecting the hypervascularity associated with this inflammatory lesion. The delayed phase (center) shows intense uptake of the radionuclide in the same distribution. A 48-hour image from a gallium scan* (right) *shows increased uptake in a similar distribution. (The increased gallium uptake indicates the inflammatory reaction within bone, whereas the positive delayed bone scan reflects the osteoblastic response.)*

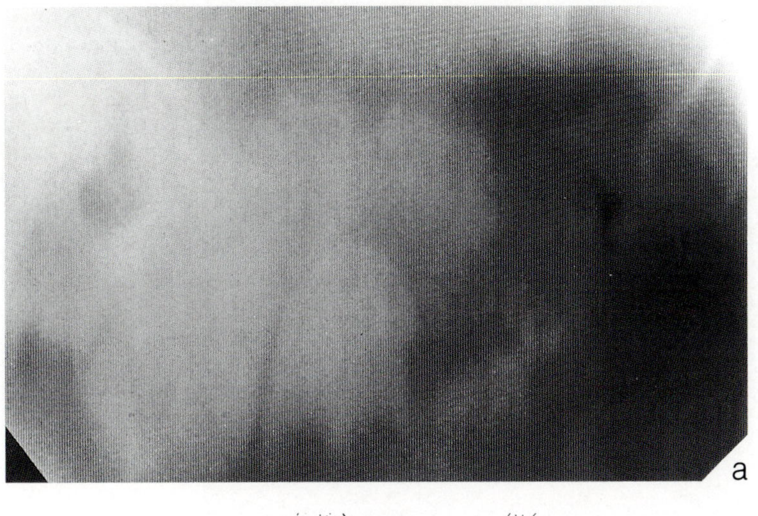

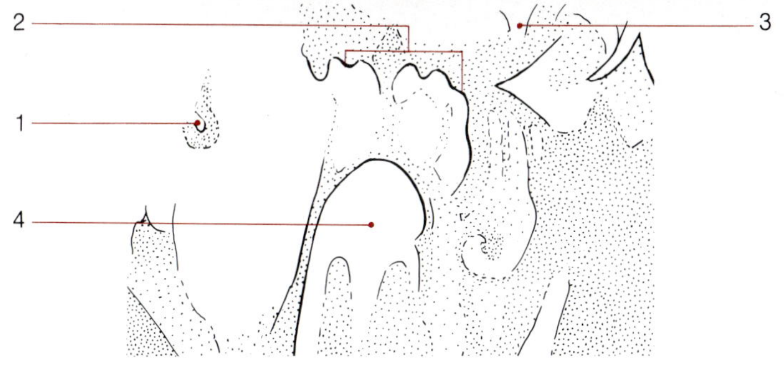

1 External auditory canal 2 Mass	3 Bone destruction in roof of glenoid fossa 4 Mandibular condyle

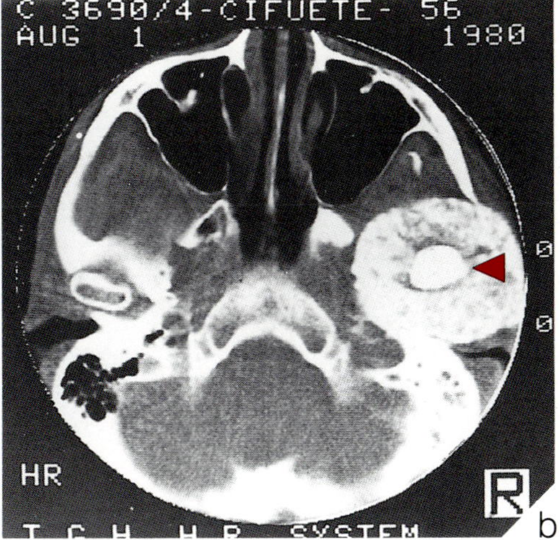

Fig. 8.2 Destructive pyrophosphate arthropathy (pseudogout) of the temporo-mandibular (TM) joint. *This 31-year-old man presented with trismus and facial swelling centered over the right TM joint. **a** A lateral complex-motion tomogram shows a large partially calcified mass within the right TM joint. The joint space is markedly expanded. The roof of the glenoid fossa has been destroyed and the calcified mass encroaches on the middle cranial fossa. The mandibular condyle is thickened and sclerotic. **b** An axial CT scan shows that the partially calcified mass expands the TM joint in all directions and encroaches on the adjacent soft tissues. The mandibular condyle (arrow) is enlarged and lacks a medullary cavity (compare with opposite side).*

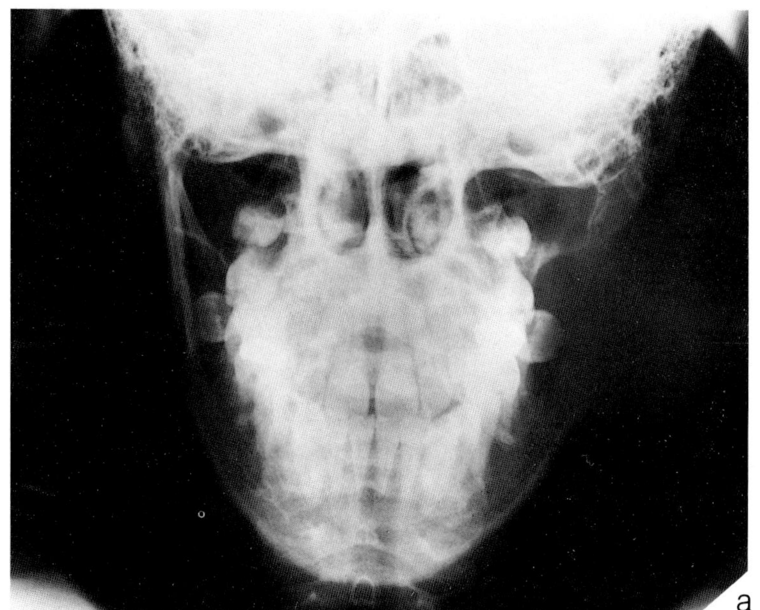

Fig. 8.3 Osteogenic sarcoma of the mandible. *This 12-year-old boy presented with a slowly enlarging painful mass in the left mandible. **a** An anteroposterior view of the mandible demonstrates a destructive lesion involving the region of the mandibular angle and most of the ramus. The cortical margin cannot be defined, suggesting that the tumor extends into the soft tissues. Compare with normal right mandible. **b** The bone scan demonstrates the extent of the tumor to better advantage.*

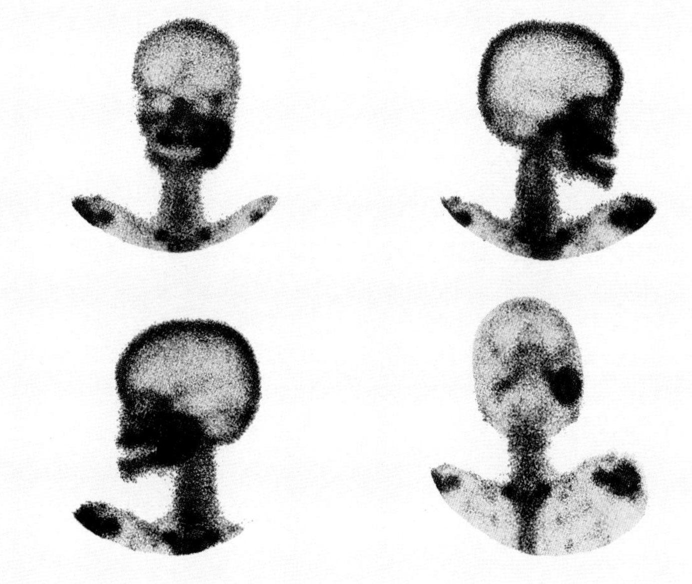

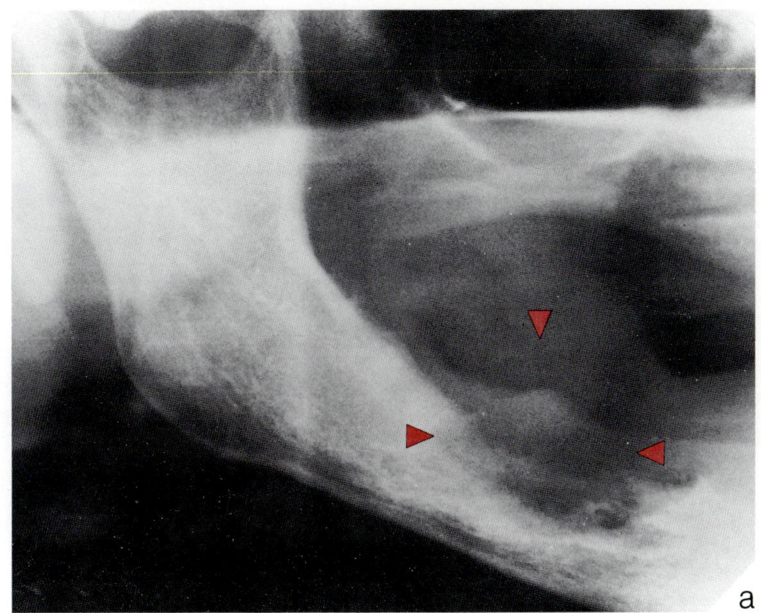

a

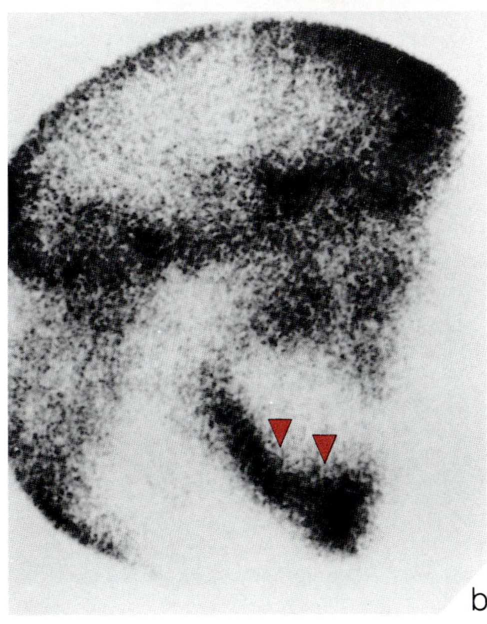

b

Fig. 8.4 Carcinoma of the oral cavity with mandibular invasion. *a In this patient with a squamous cell carcinoma originating in the floor of the mouth, a panoramic tomogram shows a localized area of bone destruction* (arrows) *in the the body of the mandible. **b** The lateral view of an MDP bone scan (delayed phase) shows the true extent of the tumor. The photon-deficient area* (arrows) *corresponds to the area of bone destruction seen on the panoramic tomogram. However, the area of increased uptake (indicating the actual extent of bone invasion) is much greater than the area of bone destruction seen radiographically. (Reproduced with permission from Noyek et al, 1987.)*

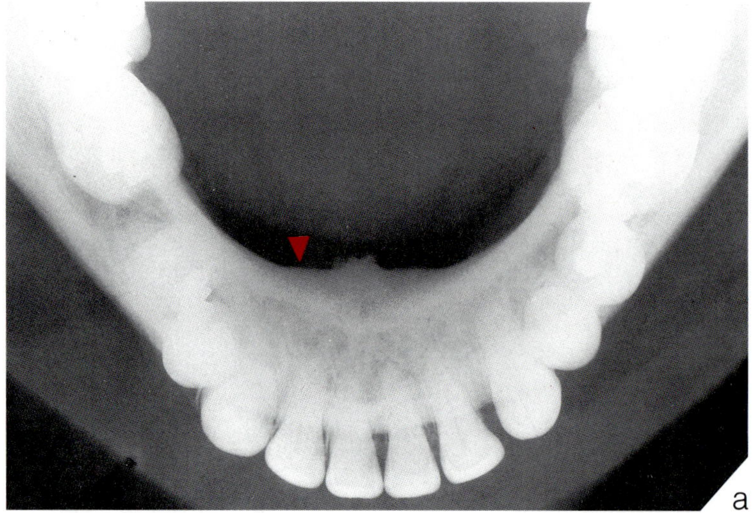

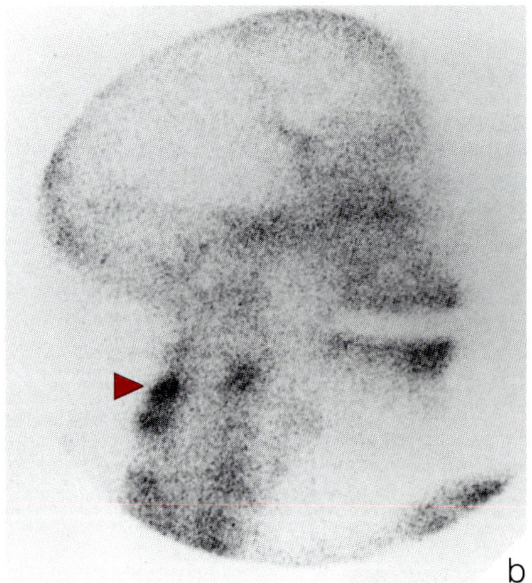

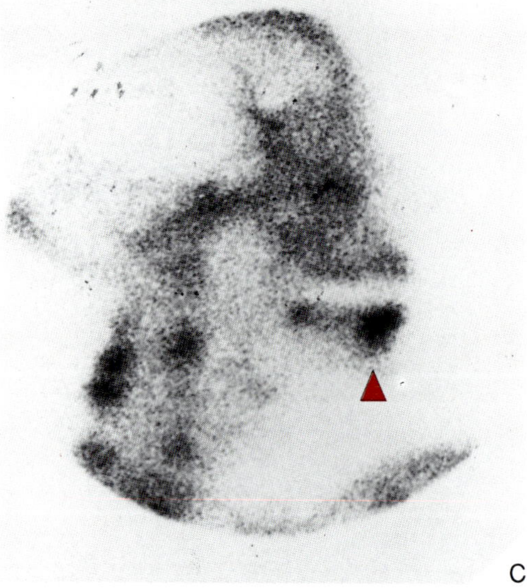

Fig. 8.5 Carcinoma of the alveolus with mandibular invasion. *This 53-year-old woman presented with a small focal squamous cell carcinoma of the alveolus. **a** A superoinferior view of the mandible obtained during the initial staging workup shows no evidence of bone abnormality. The site of the soft-tissue lesion is indicated (arrow). **b** A right lateral view of an MDP bone scan shows normal activity in the mandible, virtually excluding bone invasion. The increased uptake in the cervical spine (arrow) is due to osteoarthritis. **c** A follow-up bone scan (6 months later) shows intense focal uptake in the mandible (arrow) indicating tumor invasion. Conventional radiographs obtained at this time again showed no evidence of bone invasion.*

*M*ajor Salivary Glands

The great majority of salivary calculi occur in the submandibular gland and its duct. Whereas parotid duct stones are usually radiolucent, submandibular calculi are usually radiopaque and can be detected on plain films (Fig. 9.1). Long-standing ductal obstruction leads to acute and chronic inflammation and sialectasis.

While functional derangements of the salivary glands can be detected by radionuclide (pertechnetate) scans, contrast studies are needed to demonstrate abnormal morphology. Conventional retrograde sialography, which requires relatively large volumes of concentrated contrast medium and often causes acute sialadenitis, is

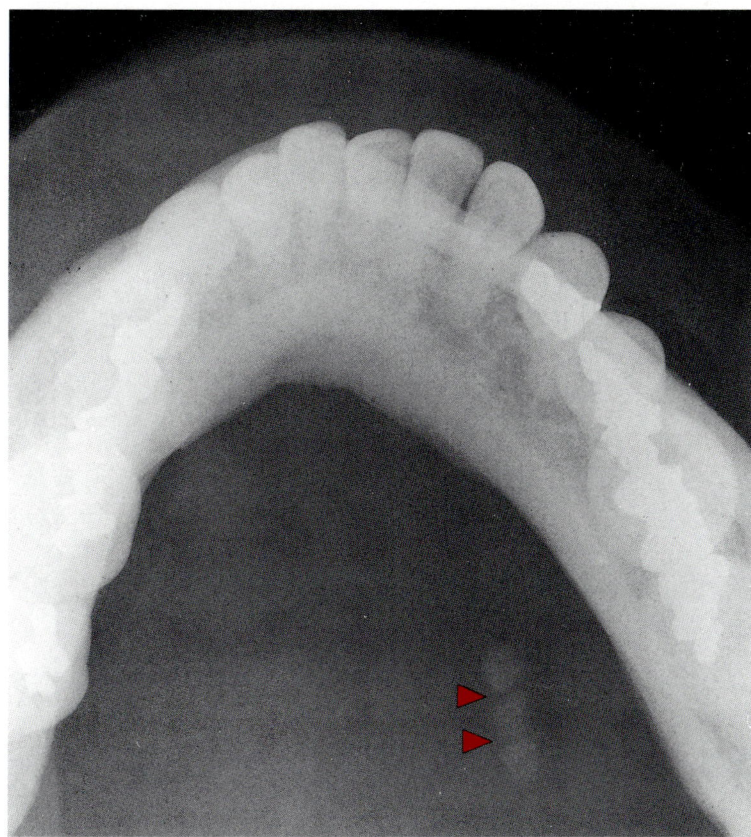

Fig. 9.1 Multiple radiopaque submandibular duct stones. *An occlusal film shows three opaque stones* (arrows) *in the left submandibular duct of a 35-year-old woman with recurrent swelling of the submandibular gland.*

seldom performed nowadays, although it remains the examination of choice in patients with known or suspected ductal stenosis (Fig. 9.2). When sialography is employed for this purpose, minimal amounts of contrast agent should be used to minimize the risk of sialadenitis. By combining sialography with CT, only small amounts of dilute water-soluble contrast agent are needed to demonstrate the intra-glandular ducts, greatly decreasing the risk of sialadenitis (Fig. 9.3).

Mass lesions of the major salivary glands are best studied by CT (Figs. 9.4–9.6). CT with contrast enhancement can detect extraparotid extension or involvement of the deep lobe or parapharyngeal space, and is routinely used to stage parotid neoplasms (Figs. 9.7, 9.8). MRI promises to revolutionize parotid imaging. One investigator

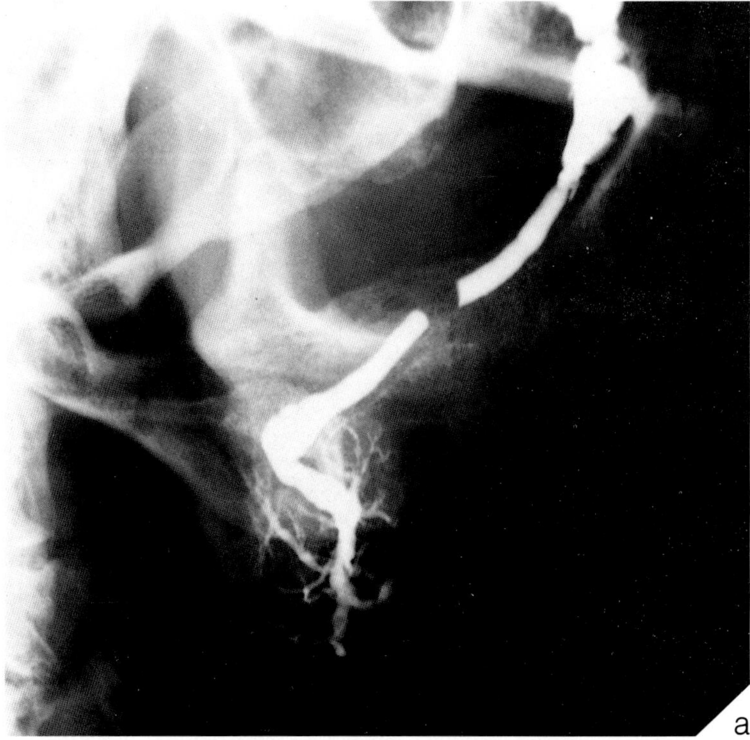

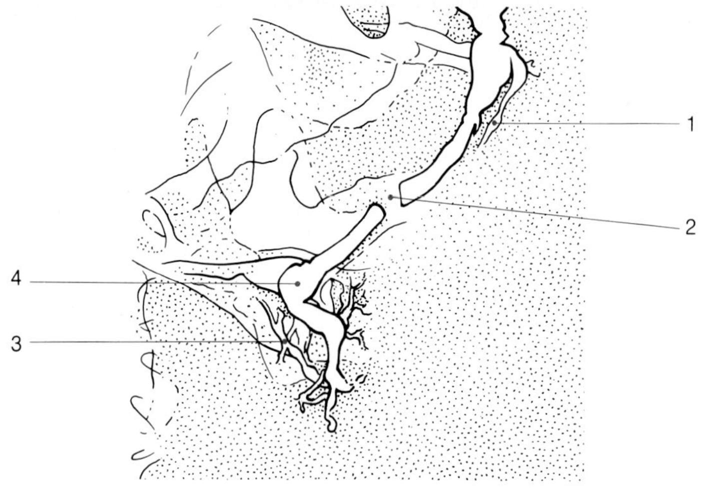

has recently published MRI scans showing the entire course of the facial nerve through the parotid gland—a "map" of inestimable value to the surgeon.

Pertechnetate scans can help define the nature of a parotid mass. A functioning ("hot") focal lesion that corresponds to the clinical mass almost invariably represents a Warthin's tumor; indeed we have yet to see a false-negative scan in this setting (see Fig. 9.3b, c). The rare oncocytoma may also appear as a "hot" lesion on the pertechnetate scan. On the other hand, a "cold" defect is of little diagnostic significance.

Technetium-pyrophosphate-tagged erythrocytes can be used to confirm the diagnosis of parotid cavernous hemangioma (Fig. 9.9).

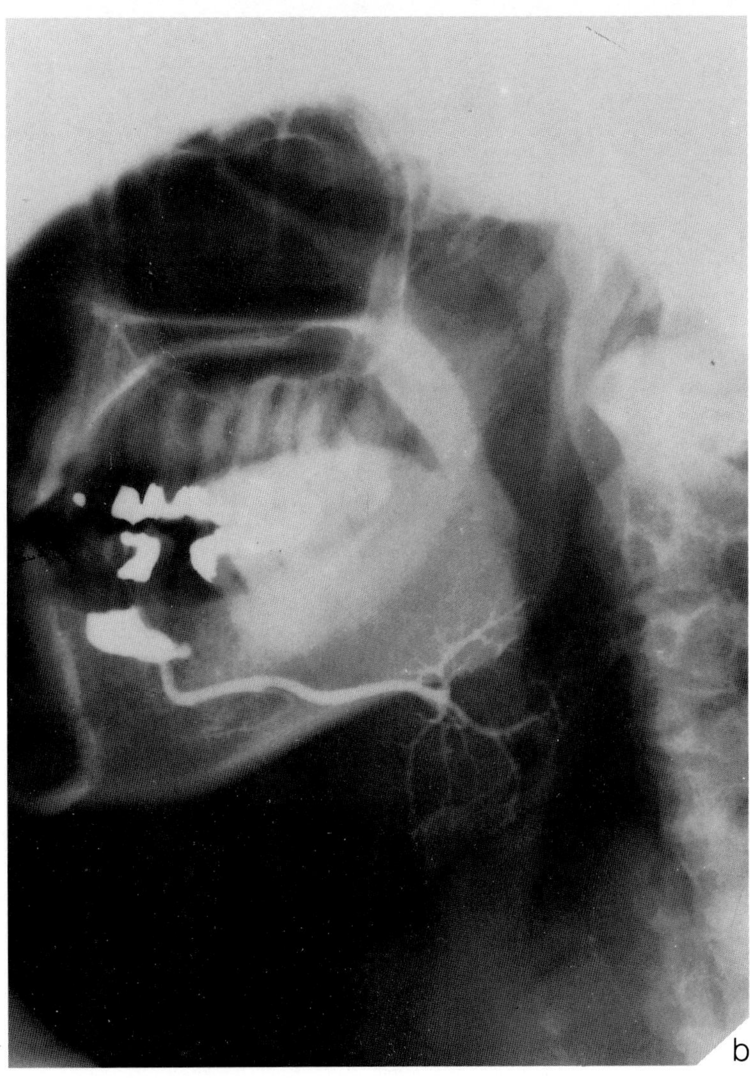

Fig. 9.2 Submandibular sialectasis; stenosis and calculus of Wharton's duct. *A 51-year-old man with recurrent submandibular swelling and pain.* ***a*** *Oblique lateral projection of a submandibular sialogram shows distention of Wharton's duct with a short stenotic segment close to the orifice; the filling defect in the duct represents a radiolucent calculus. Small intraglandular branches show beading and sacculation (sialectasis) due to chronic obstruction and inflammation.* ***b*** *Lateral projection of a normal sialogram in another patient is shown for comparison. Note uniform caliber of duct and delicate tapering pattern of intraglandular branches.*

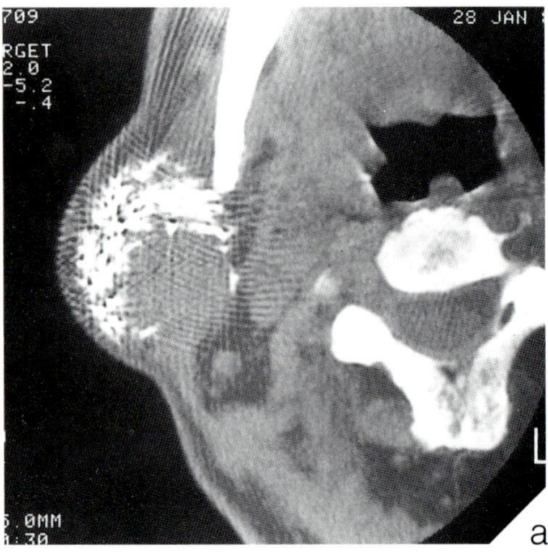
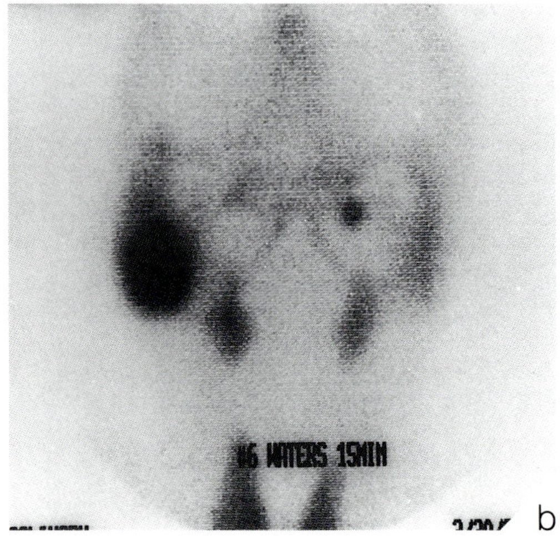
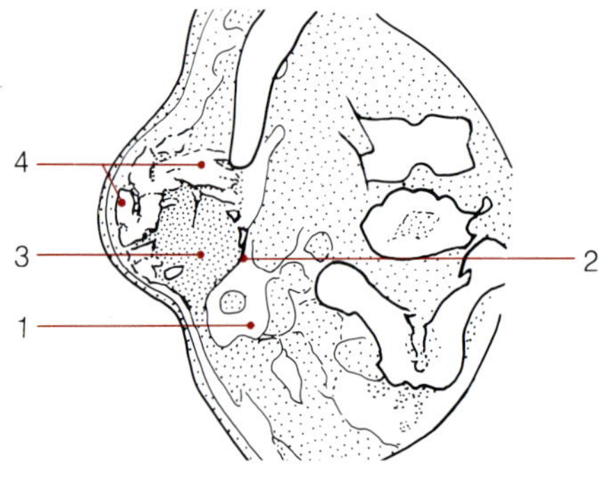
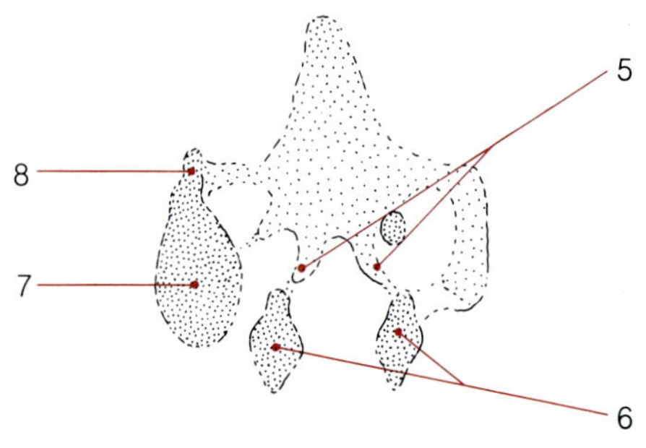

1 Normal parapharyngeal space	6 Submandibular glands
2 Deep surface of mass	7 Increased uptake in tumor
3 Mass	8 Normal portion of parotid gland
4 Normal parotid gland	9 Residual activity
5 Submandibular ducts	

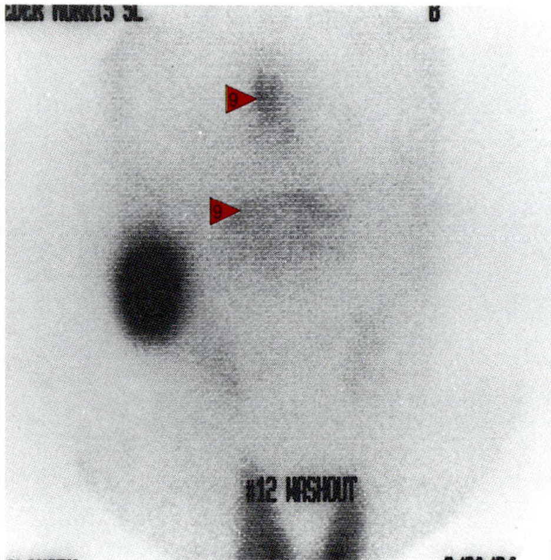

Fig. 9.3 Warthin's tumor of the parotid gland.
a An axial CT-sialogram demonstrates a mass in the right parotid gland of a 78-year-old man. Normal glandular tissue (opacified by the contrast agent) surrounds the mass. The deep surface of the parotid tumor is sharply demarcated from the fat-containing parapharyngeal space. *b* Frontal projection of a pertechnetate scan, obtained 15 minutes after bolus injection of the radionuclide, demonstrates markedly increased uptake within the parotid mass (compare with normal uptake in the other salivary glands and the unaffected peripheral portion of the right parotid gland). *c* "Washout" image obtained after administration of a sialogogue (lemon) shows persistent activity in the hyperfunctioning parotid mass. Almost all of the "hot" saliva has been excreted from the salivary apparatus into the oral cavity and swallowed; a small amount of residual activity is seen in oral and nasal secretions (arrows 9).

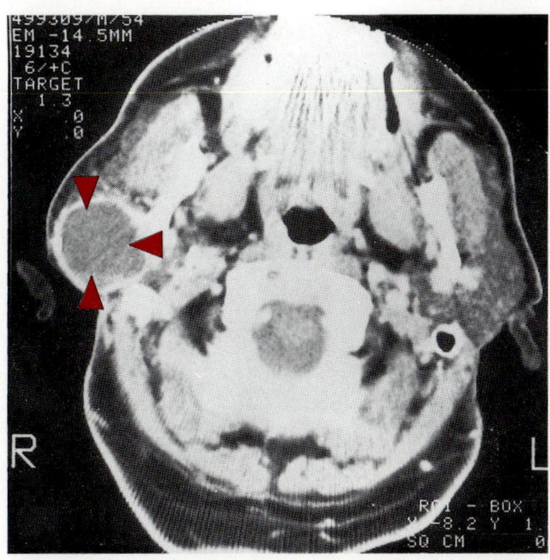

Fig. 9.4 Abscess of the parotid gland. *A contrast-enhanced axial CT scan demonstrates a large abscess cavity in the right parotid gland of a 53-year-old man. There is intense staining of the vascular abscess wall (arrows). The fluid in the dependent portion of the abscess has a relatively high CT number, consistent with fresh blood (most likely due to bleeding from a previous percutaneous aspiration).*

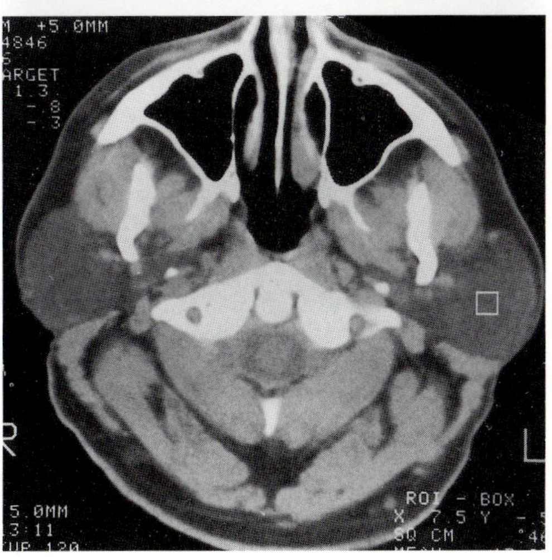

Fig. 9.5 Fatty infiltration of the parotid glands. *An axial CT scan shows massive enlargement of both parotid glands, without a discrete tumor mass in a 57-year-old diabetic man. The density (attenuation) of both parotid glands is homogeneously decreased. The mean density of the left parotid gland (measured in the region under the cursor) is -13 Hounsfield units. CT numbers in this range are compatible with fatty infiltration of the parenchyma.*

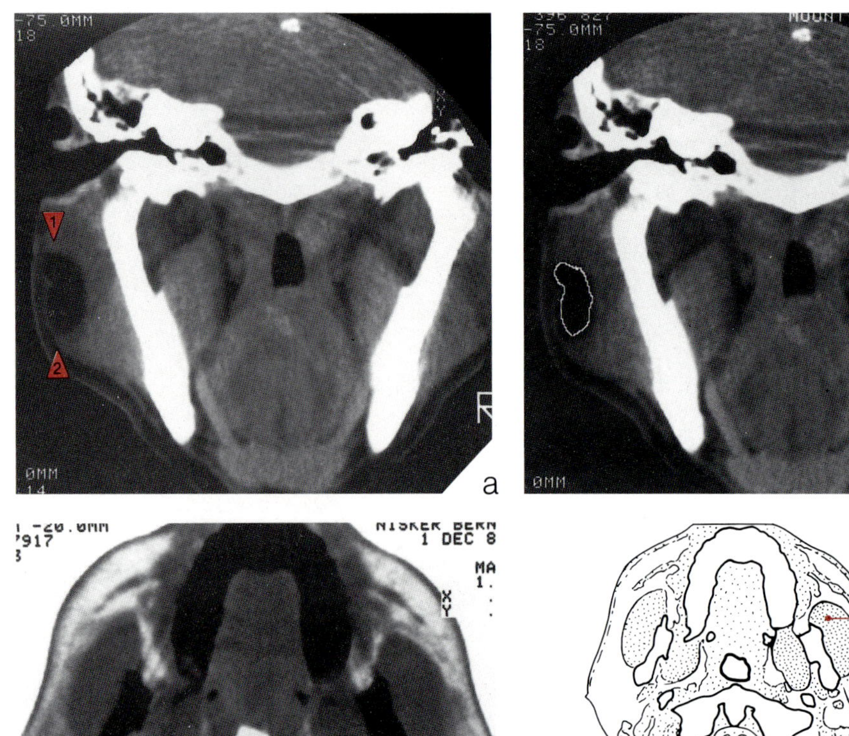
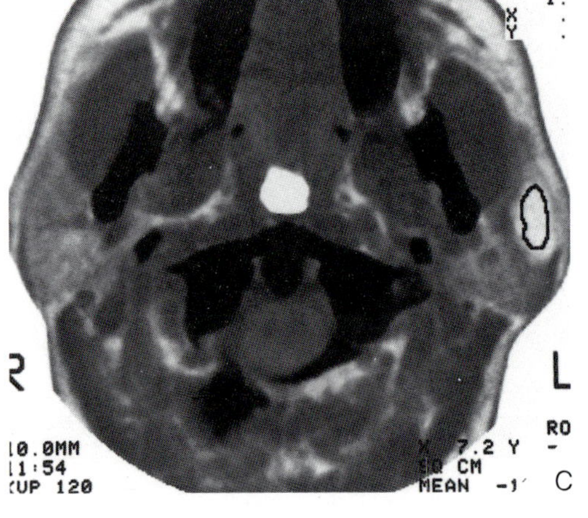

Fig. 9.6 Lipoma of the parotid gland. *This 46-year-old man presented with a parotid mass. **a** A coronal CT cut shows a low-attenuation mass within the left parotid gland. The margins of the parotid gland are indicated (arrow 1). The mass is surrounded by normal glandular tissue. The masseter muscle is indicated (arrow 2). **b** Same cut (cursor positioned over the mass) shows a mean attenuation value of -98 Hounsfield units. **c** An axial CT scan (image reversed) shows the lipoma to advantage. The mean attenuation value in the region under the cursor is -102 Hounsfield units. CT numbers in this range indicate that the mass consists entirely (or almost entirely) of fat. The margins of the parotid gland and of the masseter muscle are indicated.*

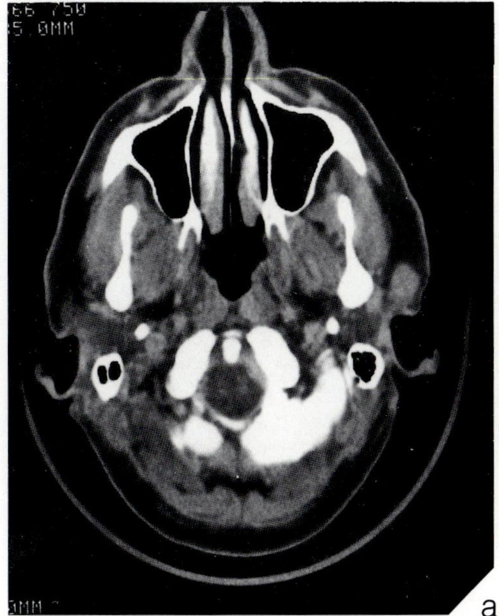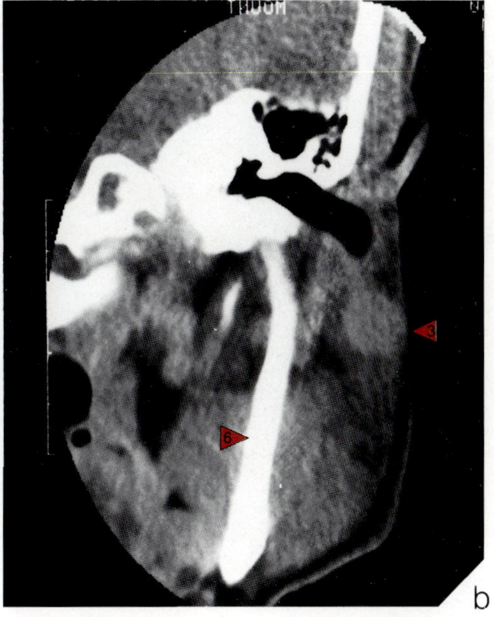

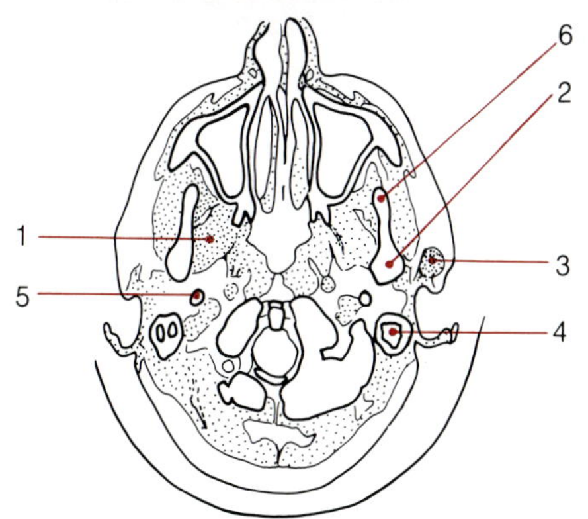

Fig. 9.7 Benign mixed tumor of the parotid gland. *a* An axial CT scan shows a well circumscribed mass (area of increased attenuation) within the left parotid gland of a 57-year-old man. *b* A coronal CT scan shows that the tumor (arrow 3) is sharply demarcated from the rest of the parotid gland and does not involve deeper structures. The mandibular ramus (arrow 6) is indicated.

1 External pterygoid muscle
2 Neck of mandible
3 Mass
4 Mastoid tip air cells
5 Styloid process
6 Mandibular ramus

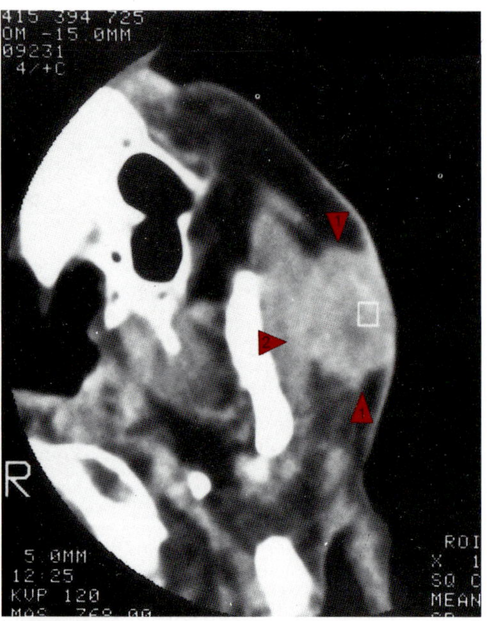

Fig. 9.8 High-grade malignant mucoepidermoid tumor of the parotid gland. *An axial CT scan shows a locally invasive tumor, marked by an irregular area of increased attenuation* (arrows 1) *arising in the left parotid gland. The tumor extends into the masseter muscle* (arrow 2), *and infiltrates the subcutaneous tissues. (Courtesy of J. Freeman, MD, Toronto Canada.)*

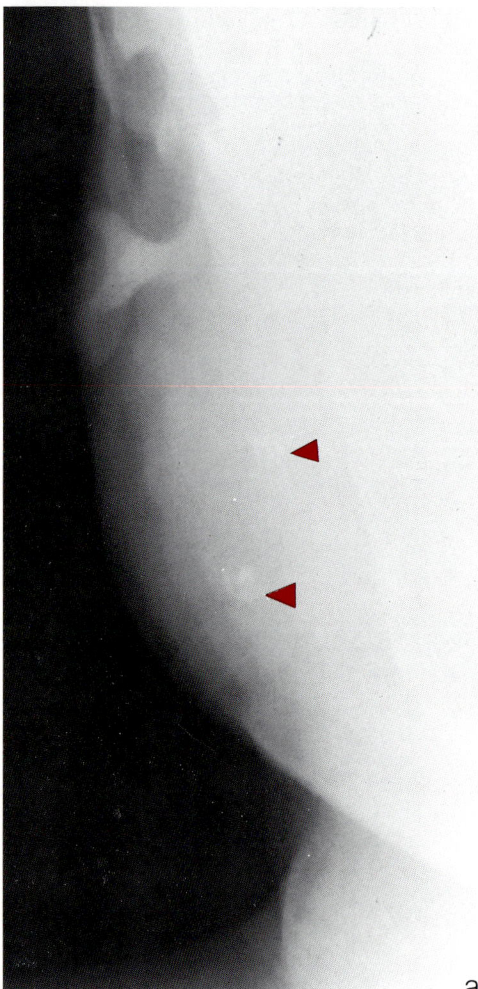

a

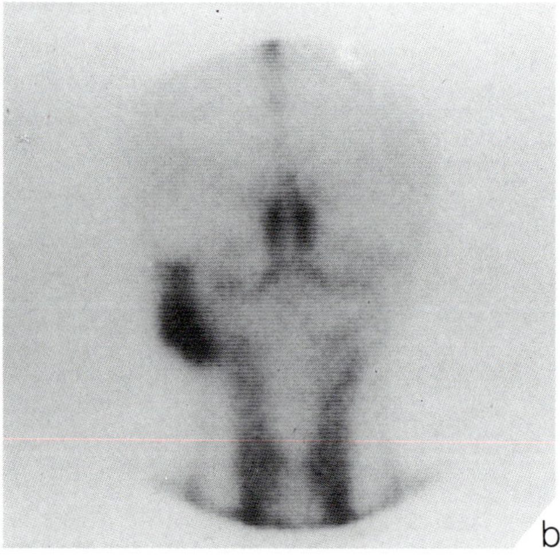

b

Fig. 9.9 Cavernous hemangioma of the parotid gland. *This 10-year-old boy presented with recurrent swelling of the right parotid gland, which was most conspicuous during exercise.* **a** *A detailed anteroposterior (AP) view of the right parotid gland shows two discrete calcifications* (arrows) *within the mass. The more caudal lesion is surrounded by a ring calcification, an appearance typical of a thrombosed phlebolith.* **b** *An anterior scintiscan obtained 50 minutes after intravenous injection of technetium 99m pyrophosphate-tagged erythrocytes shows uptake in the mass due to progressive accumulation of the tagged RBCs. These radiographic and scintigraphic findings are pathognomonic of cavernous hemangioma of the parotid gland.*

Thyroid Gland

Before the advent of high-resolution sonography, thyroid imaging was limited to radionuclide scintigraphy, which has relatively poor spatial resolution and generally cannot detect lesions under 1 cm in diameter (see Fig. 17.1). Not only can sonography detect smaller lesions than radionuclide scintigraphy, but it can differentiate cystic from nonfunctioning solid masses—both of which appear as "cold" defects on the scintiscan (Fig. 10.1). Solid lesions—even nodules only a few millimeters in diameter—are readily detected and differentiated from normal thyroid parenchyma by ultrasound. The ability to detect nodules before they can be palpated is especially important in the long-term follow-up of previously irradiated patients, who are at high risk for thyroid carcinoma (Fig. 10.2). Because of the poor resolution of pertechnetate scans, sonography is the preferred imaging technique for screening programs to detect occult thyroid disease.

Certain sonographic patterns can suggest a specific tissue diagnosis; for instance, a halo sign is characteristic of follicular adenoma. Needle aspiration of posteriorly situated or hard-to-palpate lesions can be performed under ultrasonic guidance.

The pertechnetate scan is relatively insensitive in patients with impaired thyroid function, and can be misleading in patients with thyroid masses. For definitive assessment of thyroid function (hormonogenesis), radioiodine (^{123}I) is used. The main indications for radioiodine scans are: (1) to demonstrate (or exclude) the presence of ectopic (e.g., lingual, retrosternal, or primary mediastinal) thyroid tissue; (2) to ascertain whether a "hot" nodule detected on a pertechnetate scan actually represents functioning thyroid tissue (Fig. 10.3); and (3) to demonstrate functioning metastases.

Because of its high iodine content, the thyroid gland is easily differentiated from adjacent soft tissues on CT scans. However, unless the CT examination is carefully tailored, the morphology of the gland is not well defined. The primary role of CT in thyroid imaging is to detect local extension and nodal metastases in patients with thyroid carcinoma (Figs. 10.4, 10.5). MRI may eventually prove to be very useful in evaluating benign disorders and malignancies of the thyroid gland.

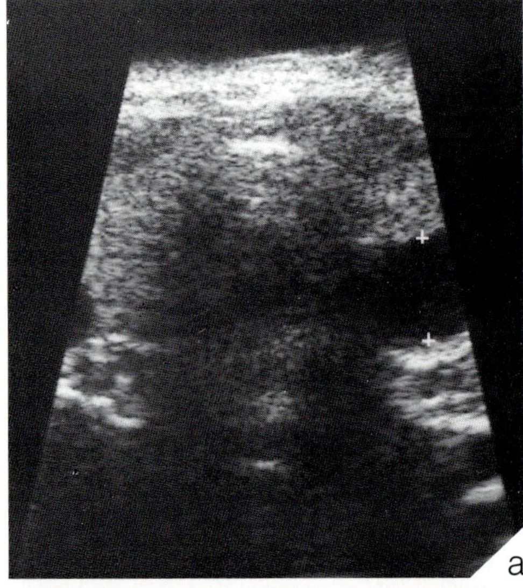

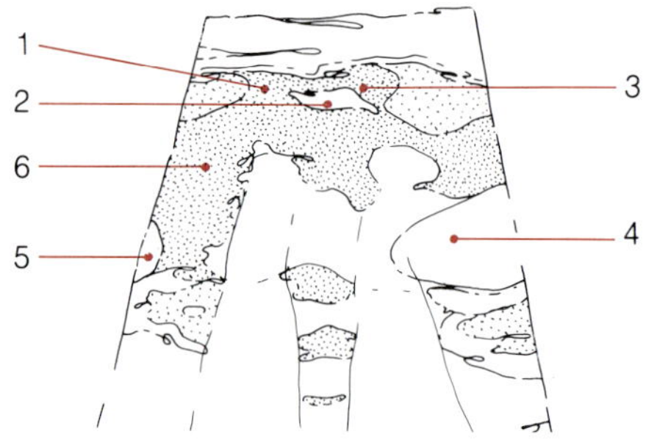

1 Strap muscles
2 Anterior wall of trachea
3 Isthmus
4 Cyst
5 Common carotid artery
6 Thyroid lobe
7 Margins of left thyroid lobe

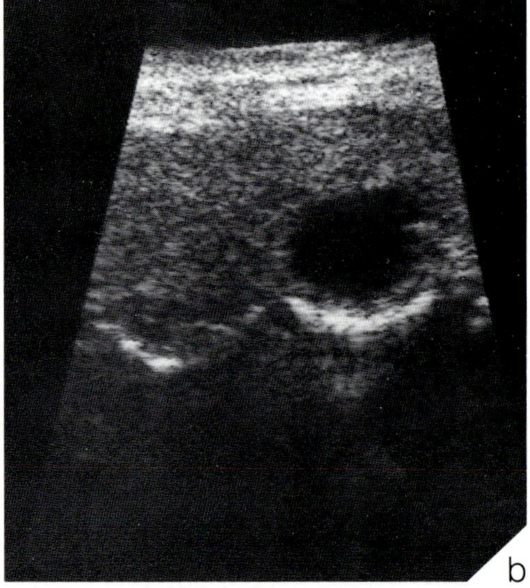

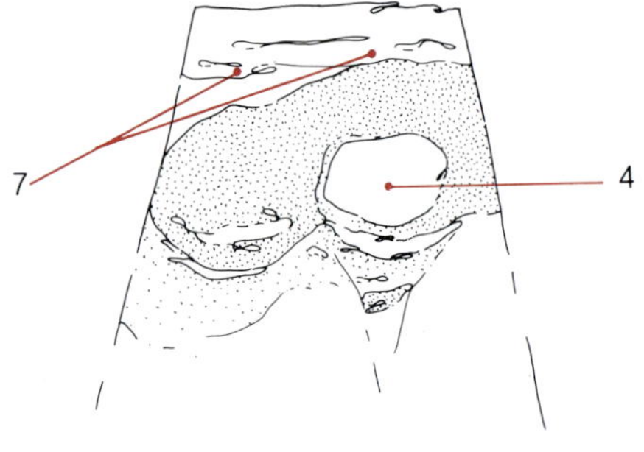

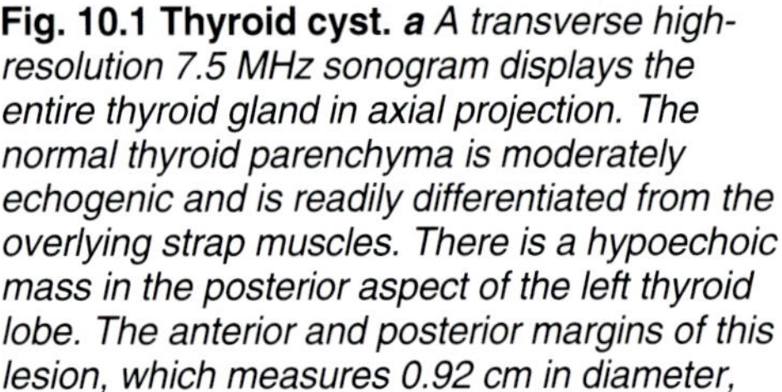

Fig. 10.1 Thyroid cyst. *a* *A transverse high-resolution 7.5 MHz sonogram displays the entire thyroid gland in axial projection. The normal thyroid parenchyma is moderately echogenic and is readily differentiated from the overlying strap muscles. There is a hypoechoic mass in the posterior aspect of the left thyroid lobe. The anterior and posterior margins of this lesion, which measures 0.92 cm in diameter, are indicated by a +. The enhanced through-transmission absence of internal echos, and strong posterior wall reverberation artifact confirm the cystic nature of the mass. **b** A parasagittal scan (longitudinal projection) shows the cyst in the inferior and posterior portion of the left thyroid lobe. The margins of the left thyroid gland are indicated.*

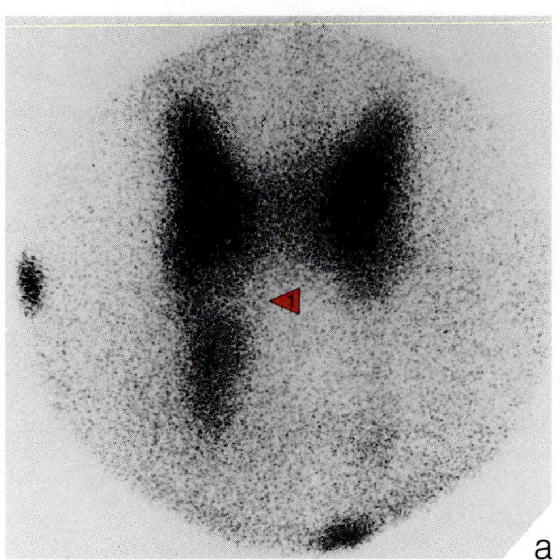

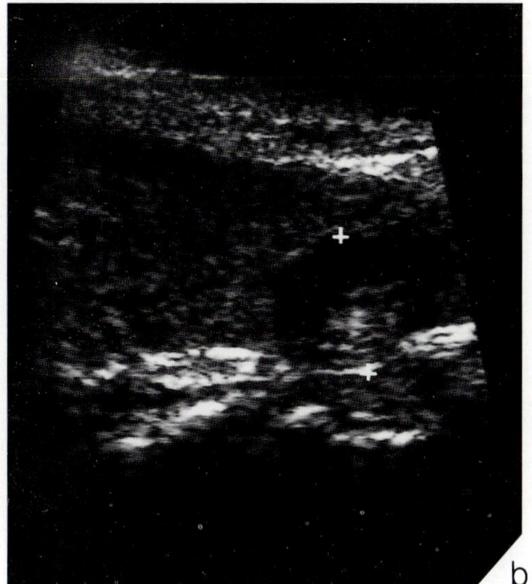

Fig. 10.2 Follicular adenoma of the thyroid gland. *This 51-year-old woman with a history of previous irradiation of the neck had a thyroid scintiscan as a routine follow-up procedure. A mass could not be palpated.* **a** *A pertechnetate scan (anterior view) shows a "cold" defect (arrow 1) in the medial aspect of the lower portion of the right thyroid lobe. The left lobe is much smaller than the right.* **b** *A high-resolution sagittal sonogram (7.5 MHz transducer) of the right thyroid lobe shows a hypoechoic focus in the posteroinferior region of the right thyroid lobe, which corresponds to the "cold" defect seen on the scintiscan. Although the lesion is predominantly cystic, a mound of echogenic tissue projects into the lumen from the posterior wall. The lesion measures 1.01 cm in diameter. Needle aspiration performed under ultrasonic guidance confirmed the diagnosis of a benign follicular adenoma.*

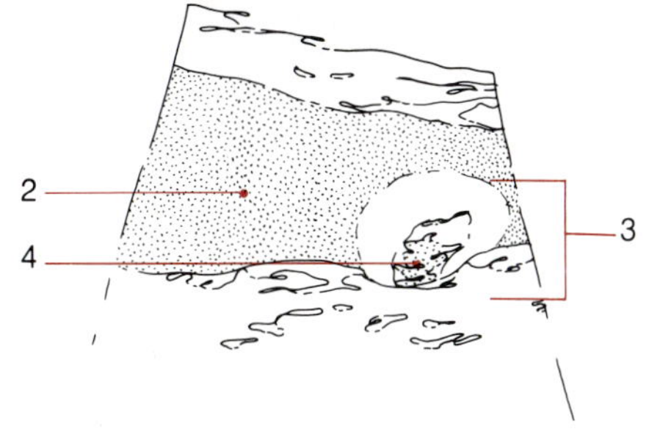

1 "Cold" defect
2 Thyroid tissue
3 Superior and inferior margins of cyst

4 Solid tissue projecting into cyst

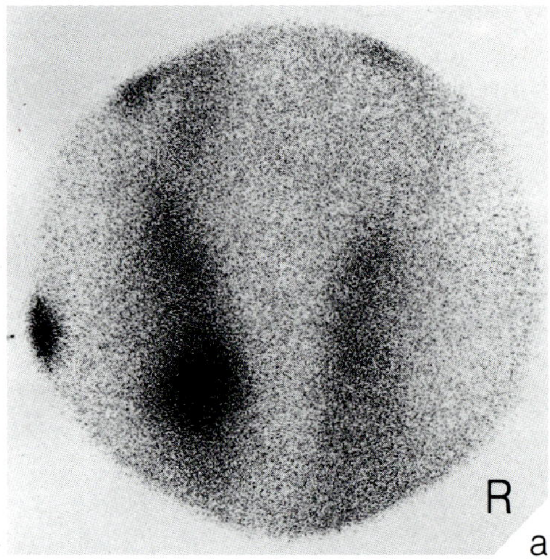

a

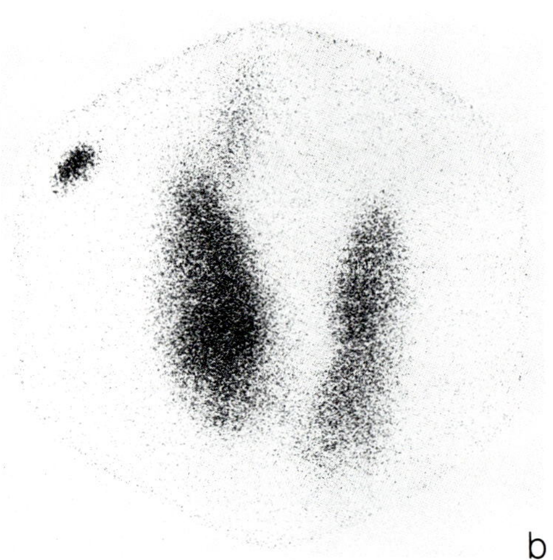
b

Fig. 10.3 False-functioning "hot" nodule (follicular adenoma). *This 56-year-old man was found to have a thyroid nodule on routine physical examination.* **a** *Anterior view of a pertechnetate thyroid scan shows an area of increased uptake ("hot" nodule) in the lower portion of the right thyroid lobe.* **b** *A ^{123}I scintiscan shows no difference in uptake between the nodule and the remainder of the right thyroid lobe. Pertechnetate uptake reflects trapping of the radionuclide by the thyroid gland whereas radioiodine uptake indicates synthesis of thyroid hormone (i.e., thyroid function). At operation the lesion proved to be a follicular adenoma.*

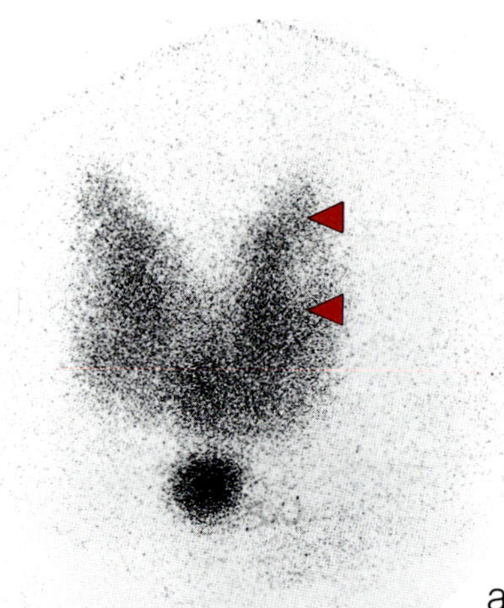
a

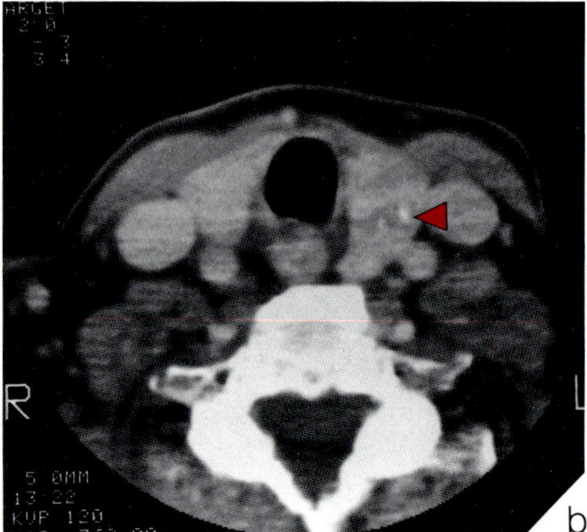

b

Fig. 10.4. Papillary carcinoma of the thyroid gland. *This 74-year-old woman presented with a thyroid nodule.* **a** *A ^{123}I thyroid scan (anterior view) demonstrates a "cold" nodule (arrows) in the upper portion of the left thyroid lobe. The "hot" spot below the thyroid is a suprasternal marker.* **b** *An axial CT scan demonstrates an irregular density within the left thyroid lobe at the level of the lesion seen on the radionuclide scan. The lesion contains a single area of calcification (arrow) and is not sharply demarcated from normal thyroid tissue. At operation this proved to be a papillary carcinoma with extracapsular extension.*

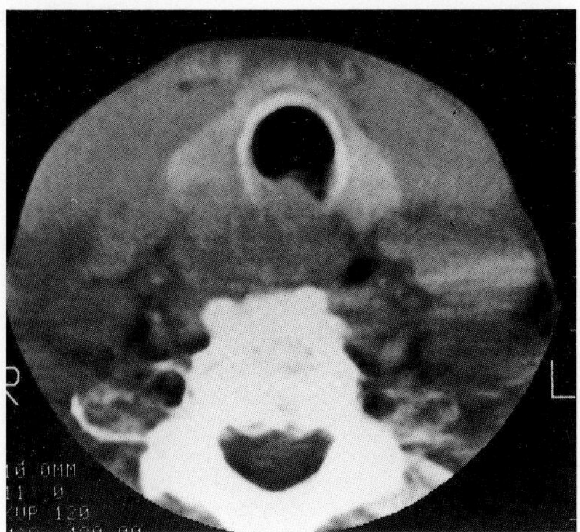

Fig. 10.5 Carcinoma of the larynx invading the thyroid gland. *An axial CT scan of a patient with a locally invasive carcinoma of the larynx shows a bulky tumor mass posterior to the trachea. The tumor has invaded the posterior portion of the right thyroid lobe (compare with uninvolved portion of thyroid gland, which has a relatively high CT number owing to its iodine content). The tumor also extends into the posterior aspect of the trachea. (Reproduced with permission from Rothberg et al, 1986.)*

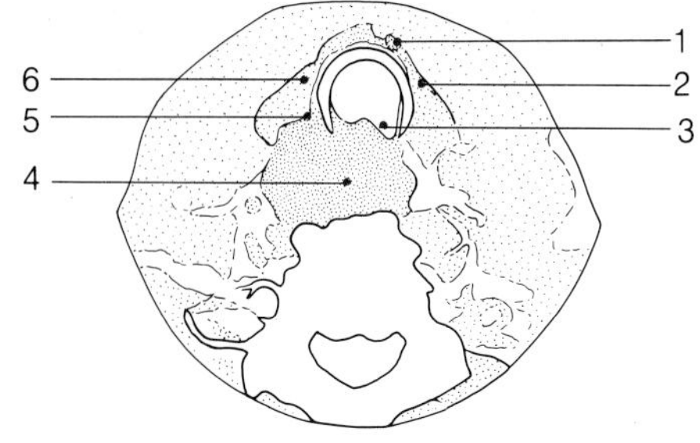

1	Thyroid isthmus	4	Tumor
2	Left thyroid lobe	5	Invasion of posterior portion of right thyroid lobe
3	Tumor extension into posterior aspect of trachea	6	Normal portion of right thyroid lobe

Parathyroid Gland

Neck exploration by an experienced parathyroid surgeon will cure the hypercalcemia in more than 90 percent of patients with presumptive biochemical evidence of hyperparathyroidism; thus the precise role for preoperative parathyroid localization is unclear. Most surgeons agree that preoperative localization is helpful in patients who have undergone a previous negative neck exploration and continue to be symptomatic (presumably due to an adenoma in an ectopic location), and in high-risk patients in whom preoperative localization might minimize the time spent under anesthesia. I believe successful preoperative imaging of an adenoma decreases surgical morbidity, such as hypocalcemia.

Because of their small size (generally 5 mm or less at greatest dimension, with an average weight of 35 to 40 mg), normal parathyroid glands are seldom demonstrated on CT or sonography. Markedly enlarged glands (500 mg or more) can be detected by various noninvasive techniques, including high-resolution ultrasound (Figs. 11.1, 11.2), thallium/technetium pertechnetate computer-generated subtraction scintigraphy, and dynamic CT scans, in which serial images are obtained at preselected levels following intravenous adminis-tration of a bolus of contrast material. A "positive" CT scan must be interpreted with caution, as a tortuous vessel, a collapsed esophagus, a thyroid mass, or a lymph node can be mistaken for an enlarged parathyroid gland. Noninvasive imaging techniques have generally been unrewarding in patients with small adenomas or mild to moderate four-gland hyperplasia. Whether MRI will be more informative than currently available imaging techniques remains to be seen; my preliminary experience suggests that it is superb in adenoma identification.

Angiographic localization techniques, such as selective parathyroid arteriography (SPA) and venous sampling, are generally reserved for patients who have undergone unsuccessful parathyroid surgery. In one recent study, 85 percent of abnormal glands were detected by SPA. Because SPA requires considerable expertise and carries a significant risk of stroke or spinal cord infarction, it is performed in only a few centers. Recent studies suggest that abnormal parathyroid glands can be located by digital subtraction angiography (DSA) in as many as half the cases, eliminating the need for SPA.

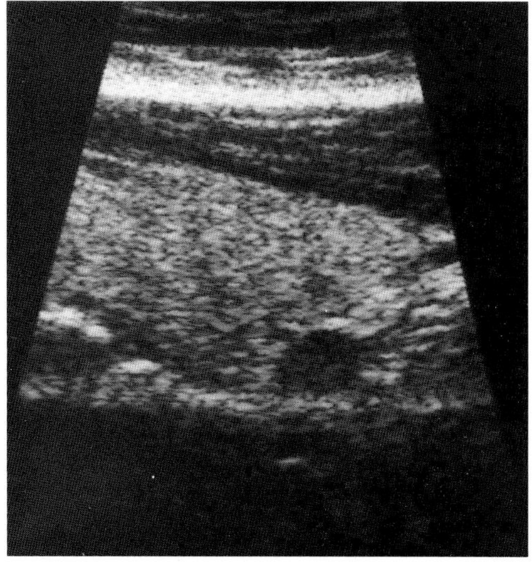

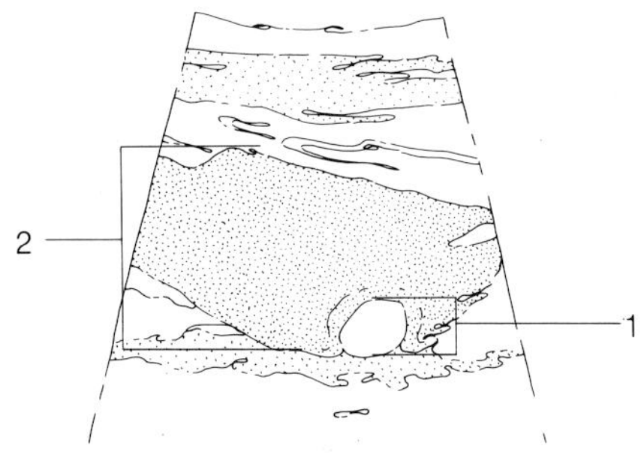

| 1 Parathyroid-adenoma | 2 Margins of left thyroid lobe |

Fig. 11.1 Parathyroid adenoma. *A high-resolution sonogram in a patient with primary hyperparathyroidism shows a hypoechoic lesion (parathyroid adenoma) indenting the posteroinferior surface of the left thyroid lobe. The margins of the left thyroid lobe are indicated. The lesion measures 0.8 cm in diameter.*

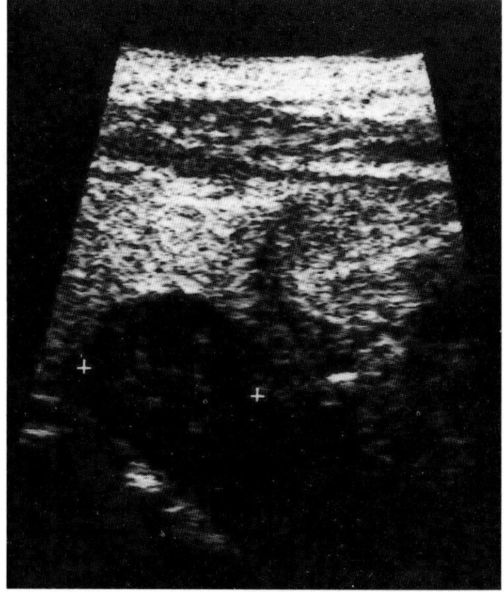

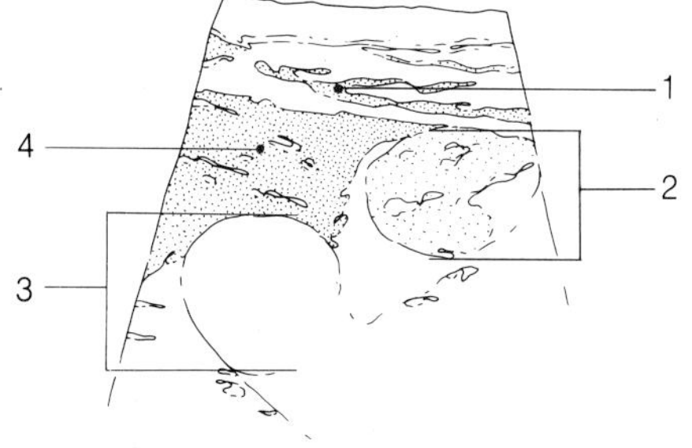

| 1 Strap muscles | 3 Parathyroid adenoma |
| 2 Follicular adenoma | 4 Normal thyroid tissue |

Fig. 11.2 Parathyroid adenoma and thyroid follicular adenoma. *A parasagittal high-resolution sonogram in a 37-year-old man who presented with hypercalcemia shows a large hypoechoic mass (parathyroid adenoma) posterior to the left thyroid lobe, in the position of the left superior parathyroid gland. The mass measures 15 mm in longitudinal dimension. Also noted is an echogenic mass within the lower portion of the left thyroid lobe. The mass, which proved at operation to be a follicular adenoma, has a relatively hypoechoic border (halo sign), a finding commonly associated with this lesion.*

Superior Mediastinum

The superior mediastinum is of interest to the oto-laryngologist, as mass lesions arising in the neck can extend into this anatomic region, affecting structures that traverse the thoracic inlet. Conventional chest films or tomograms often demonstrate the mediastinal mass (Fig. 12.1), though subtle displacement and/or compression of the trachea may be the only radiographic finding in some instances. A barium swallow may reveal displacement, narrowing, or obstruction of the esophagus. In general, CT or MRI is needed for accurate localization and characterization of neck masses that extend into the mediastinum (Fig. 12.2). Radionuclide scintigraphy is useful in spe-cific circumstances. For example, a pertechnetate or radioiodine scan may confirm the diagnosis of retrosternal or mediastinal thyroid (see Fig. 12.1b), while gallium citrate scans play an important role in the preliminary staging of lymphoma.

Superior mediastinal masses commonly distort vascular anatomy and prior knowledge of the altered relations may be of great help to the surgeon. DSA provides a satisfactory display of the great vessels from the level of the aortic arch cephalad, often eliminating the need for more invasive angiographic procedures (see Fig. 12.1d).

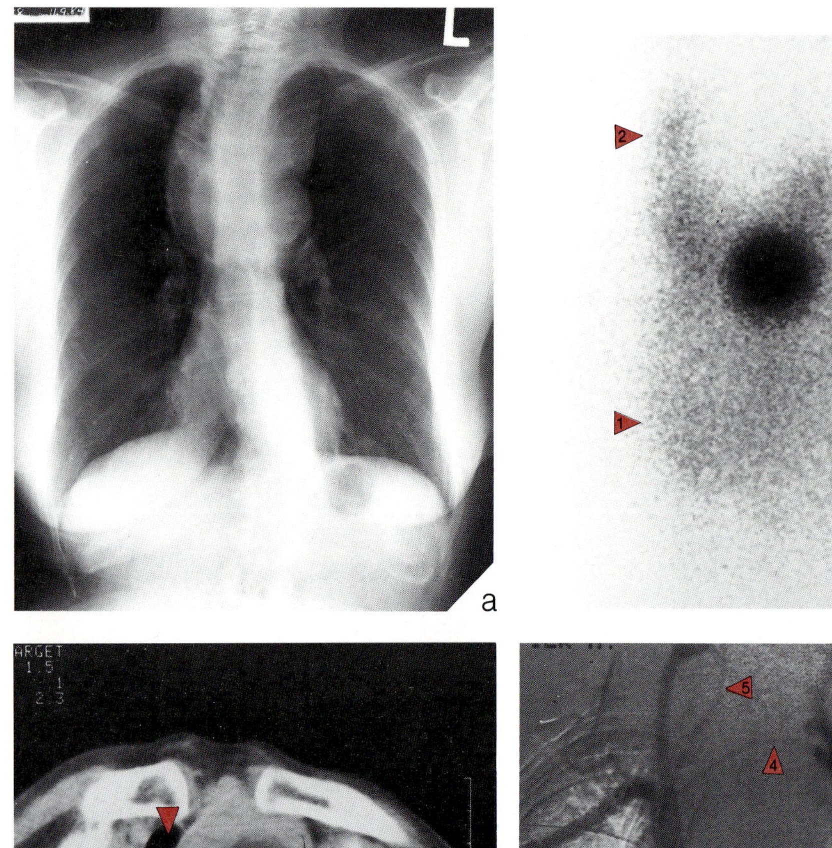

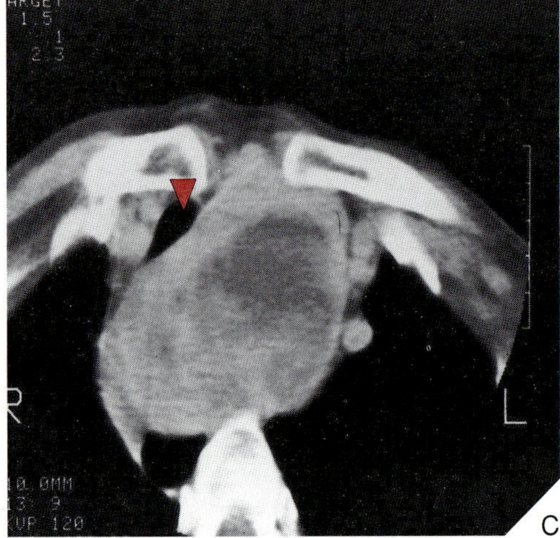

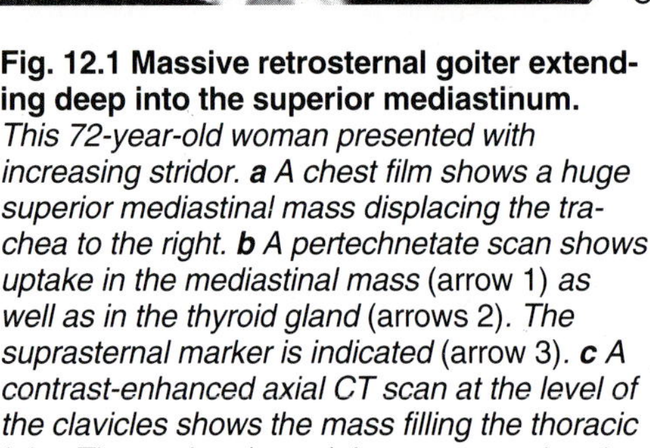

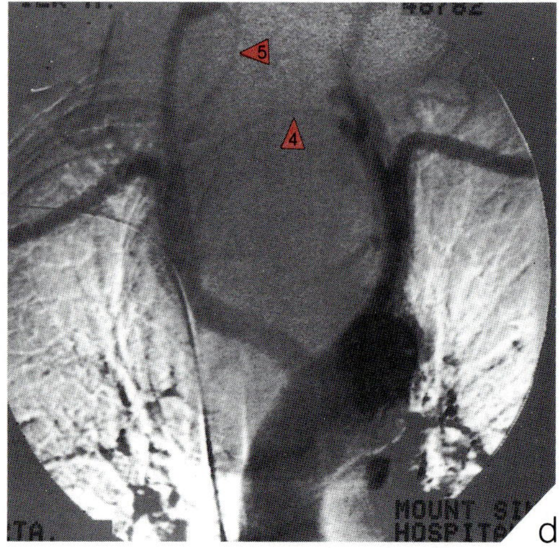

Fig. 12.1 Massive retrosternal goiter extending deep into the superior mediastinum.
*This 72-year-old woman presented with increasing stridor. **a** A chest film shows a huge superior mediastinal mass displacing the trachea to the right. **b** A pertechnetate scan shows uptake in the mediastinal mass (arrow 1) as well as in the thyroid gland (arrows 2). The suprasternal marker is indicated (arrow 3). **c** A contrast-enhanced axial CT scan at the level of the clavicles shows the mass filling the thoracic inlet. The trachea (arrow) is compressed and displaced to the right. The large areas of decreased attenuation within the mass suggest that it is a colloid goiter. **d** DSA shows that the blood supply of the mass comes from the left inferior thyroid artery (arrow 4), a branch of the thyrocervical trunk, and the right superior thyroid artery (arrow 5), a branch of the external carotid artery. None of the blood supply comes from below. Because the blood supply of this huge mass is derived entirely from vessels in the neck, I was able to resect it through a cervical approach.*

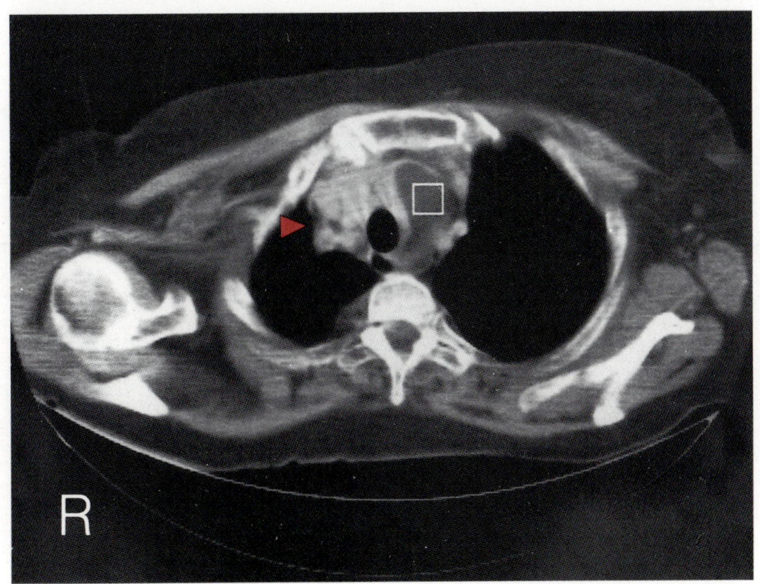

Fig. 12.2 Thyroid cyst extending into the superior mediastinum. *This 88-year-old woman presented with a mass in the left thyroid lobe and a recurrent laryngeal nerve paralysis. An axial CT scan at the level of the upper sternum demonstrates a cystic mass in the lower pole of the left thyroid lobe, which extends retrosternally (the tip of the lower pole of the right thyroid lobe (arrow) is also seen in this cut). The cyst contents have a mean attenuation number of -17 Hounsfield units; CT numbers of -20 to +20 Hounsfield units indicate water or "water-density" material (e.g., serous effusions or cyst contents).*

*L*arynx and Cervical Trachea

The larynx is readily accessible to direct inspection by conventional mirror examination, rigid and flexible telescopes, and endoscopy. However, certain structures—the ventricles and subglottic segment in particular—are difficult to visualize, and the laryngeal framework itself is quite inaccessible.

Plain films provide an overview of the larynx, and are very informative in patients with acute or chronic upper airway obstruction (Fig. 13.1), laryngeal foreign bodies, or major traumatic injuries (Fig. 13.2). Frontal and lateral projections should always be obtained when a laryngeal foreign body is suspected. Because overlying bony structures often obscure soft-tissue detail, the upper airway may be difficult to evaluate on the frontal projection; this problem can be overcome by using a copper or Thoreus filter to harden the beam. Although plain films are useful in the initial management of laryngeal injuries, CT is needed for definitive assessment.

Other conventional radiographic techniques include fluoroscopy, tomography, and contrast laryngography. Air-filled laryngoceles are easily diagnosed by fluoroscopy or conventional tomography in the coronal plane (Fig. 13.3). (The fluid-filled laryngocele, which can mimic a tumor, is more elusive and CT may be needed to confirm the diagnosis.) Once the mainstay of pretreatment tumor staging, the contrast laryngogram has been almost entirely supplanted by CT and MRI.

CT plays a crucial role in the management of laryngeal cancer, both to document the extent of advanced laryngeal cancer and to accurately stage any tumor whose accurate boundaries cannot be established clinically or endoscopically. The latter include squamous cell carcinomas arising in the supraglottic, glottic, and subglottic regions; marginal carcinomas of the aryepiglottic fold; and primary malignancies of the postcricoid region and piriform sinus. By detecting invasion of the thyroid and cricoid cartilages, as well as subglottic extension, CT allows accurate T staging prior to treatment in patients with advanced glottic and transglottic cancer (Figs. 13.4, 13.5). CT can also detect nodal metastases that are not apparent clinically, increasing the precision of N staging as well.

High-resolution thin-section MRI using shaped radiofrequency coils demonstrates the normal and abnormal larynx in exquisite detail; several studies have shown that cartilage invasion is beautifully demonstrated by MRI (Fig. 13.6). As this new modality becomes more widely available, it can be expected to join CT as the "gold standard" for staging laryngeal neoplasms.

Certain benign lesions of the larynx (e.g., arteriovascular malformations) can be accurately characterized by CT, avoiding the need for more invasive procedures (Fig. 13.7).

The imaging techniques described above can also be used to assess the subglottic larynx and cervical trachea. The sequelae of blunt and surgical trauma (e.g., subglottic or tracheal stenosis) are the most frequent indications for radiologic evaluation of this region. Primary tumors of the cervical trachea are rare (Fig. 13.8); however, secondary invasion of the cervical trachea by another malignancy is not uncommon (see Fig. 11.1). Extrinsic displacement and/or compression of the cervical trachea is usually due to a mass arising in the thyroid gland (see Figs. 12.1, 12.2) or the superior mediastinum.

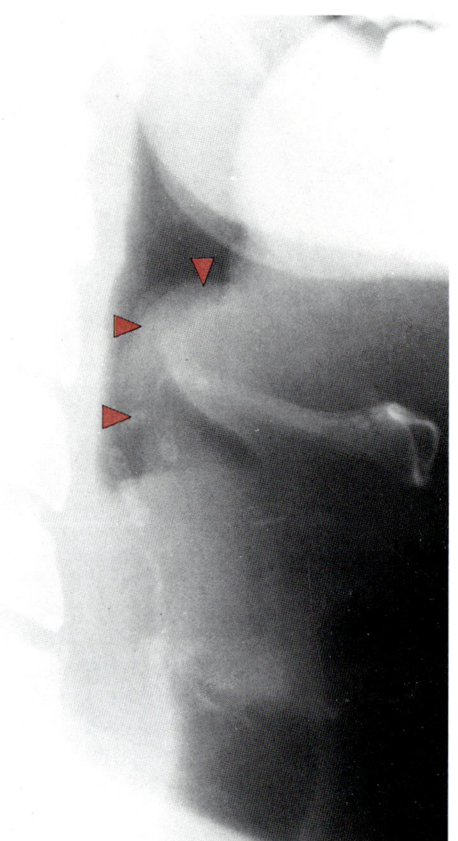

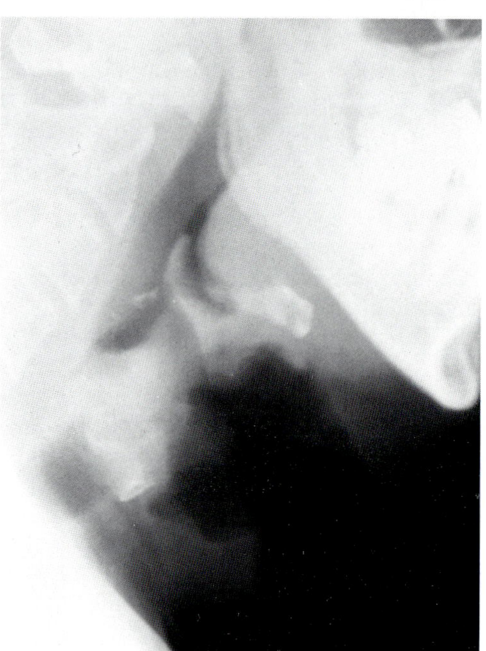

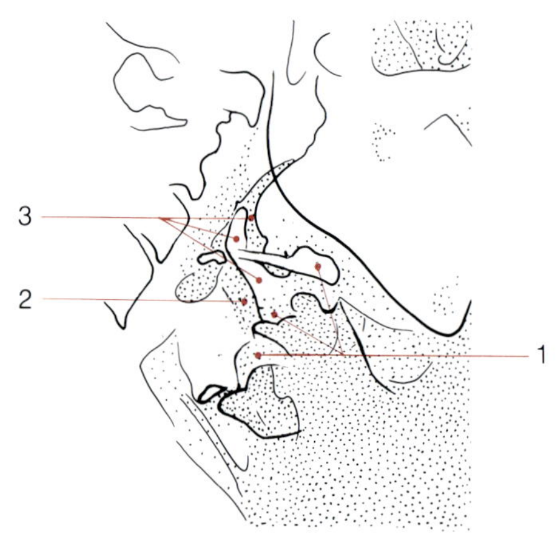

| 1 Disruption of superficial soft tissue | 2 Petiolus |
| 3 Epiglottis |

Fig. 13.1 Acute epiglottitis. *A soft-tissue lateral radiograph in a 22-year-old man with a sore throat and "air hunger" shows marked swelling of the epiglottis (arrows). (Compare with normal epiglottis in Fig. 13.2) (Note: The diagnosis of acute epiglottitis should be established as quickly as possible, as immediate control of the airway by means of endotracheal intubation or tracheostomy may be lifesaving. Indirect laryngography is sometimes technically difficult— and may sometimes be hazardous—in patients with acute epiglottitis. However, a lateral radiograph, which is nearly always diagnostic, can often be obtained with little risk to the patient.)*

Fig. 13.2 Laryngeal trauma. *A lateral radiograph in a man with a self-inflicted stab wound of the neck shows disruption of the superficial soft tissues. The base of the epiglottis has been transected from its attachment at the petiolus.*

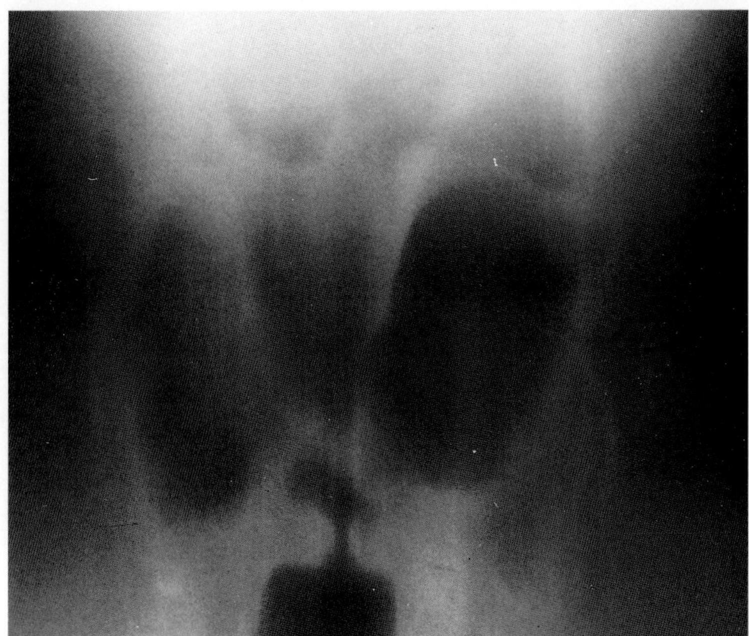

Fig. 13.3 Internal laryngocele. *An anteroposterior tomogram in a 71-year-old man shows a large air sac (obstructed internal laryngocele) on the left. The laryngocele originates in the left laryngeal ventricle, which is partially obliterated, and encroaches on the left piriform sinus.*

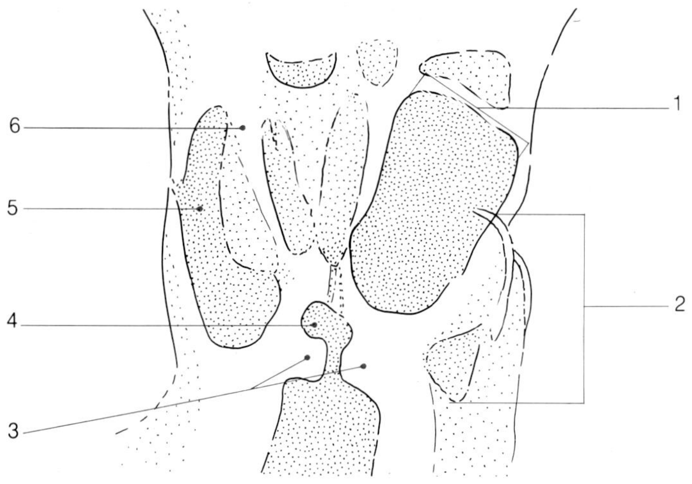

1 Laryngocele	4 Ventricle	
2 Piriform sinus	5 Piriform sinus	
3 Vocal cords	6 Right aryepiglottic fold	

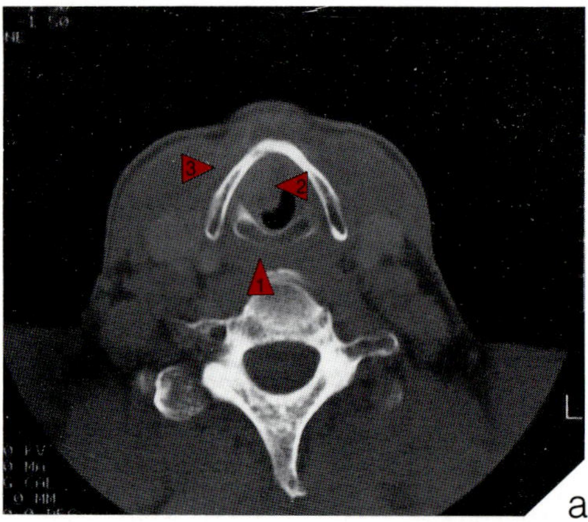
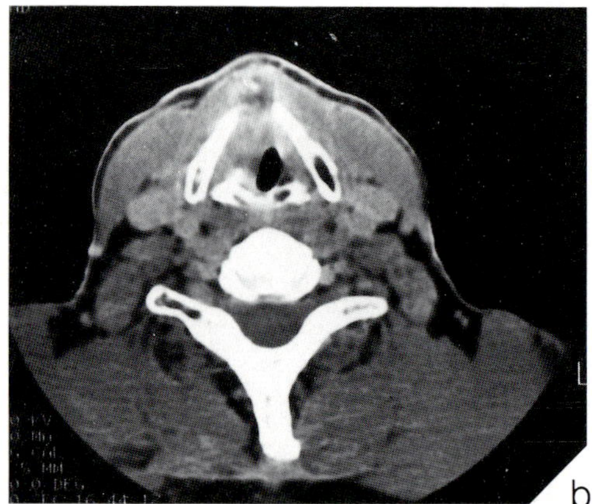
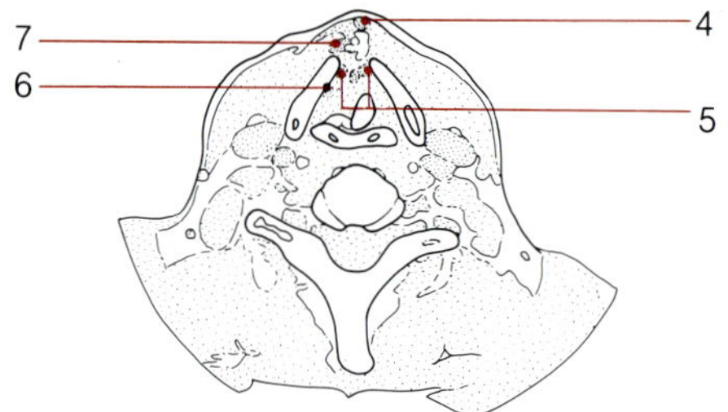

Fig. 13.4 Carcinoma of the larynx with subglottic and extralaryngeal extension (T4).
a An axial CT scan at the level of the posterior lamina of the cricoid cartilage (arrow 1) shows subglottic extension of an intralaryngeal tumor mass—squamous cell carcinoma (arrow 2). The thyroid cartilage is indicated (arrow 3). b A cut through the glottis (about 1 cm cephalad to a) shows necrotic tumor extending anteriorly into the soft tissues of the neck. The central portion of the thyroid cartilage has been destroyed. The tumor encroaches on the airway and has obliterated the anterior commissure. The patient is a 58-year-old man.

1 Cricoid cartilage
2 Squamous cell carcinoma
3 Thyroid cartilage
4 Anterior extent of tumor
5 Cartilage destruction
6 Tumor
7 Necrotic tumor

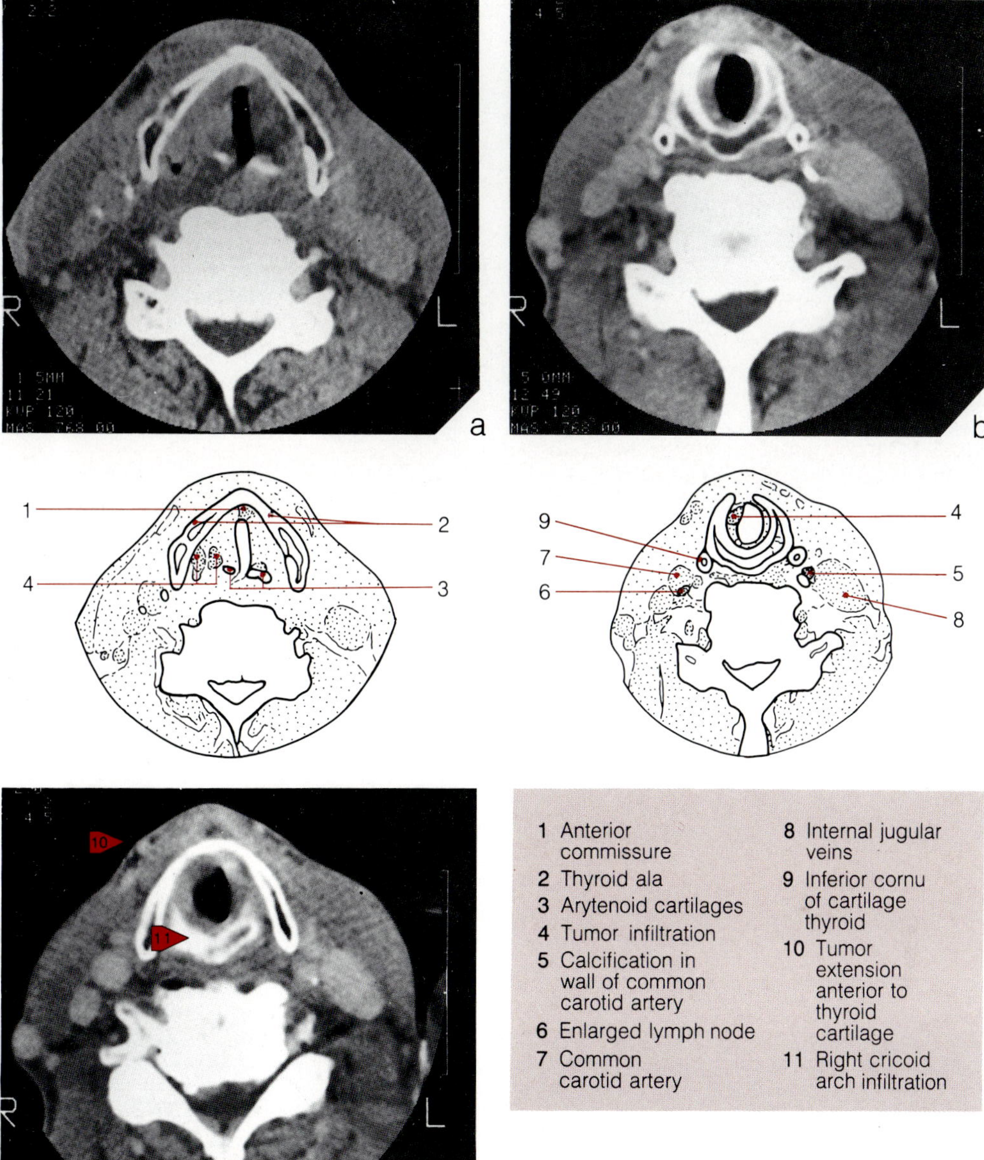

Fig. 13.5 Carcinoma of the larynx with extralaryngeal extension (T4). *A 65-year-old man with a locally advanced squamous cell carcinoma. **a** An axial CT cut at the level of the arytenoid cartilages shows obliteration of the anterior commissure by the tumor which infiltrates posteriorly between the right arytenoid cartilage and the right thyroid ala (compare normal interval between the arytenoid cartilage and the thyroid ala on the left). **b** An axial cut (with contrast enhancement) through the subglottic segment demonstrates annular submucosal infiltration by the tumor. The nonenhancing structure between the right internal jugular vein and common carotid artery is an enlarged lymph node presumably representing a metastasis. The left internal jugular vein is considerably larger than the right, a normal variant. **c** A slightly higher axial scan shows circumferential constriction of the airway by the tumor, which extends into the soft tissues anterior to the thyroid cartilage (arrow 10). The right cricoid arch is infiltrated by tumor (arrow 11) and appears more dense than the normal marrow-containing cricoid arch on the left.*

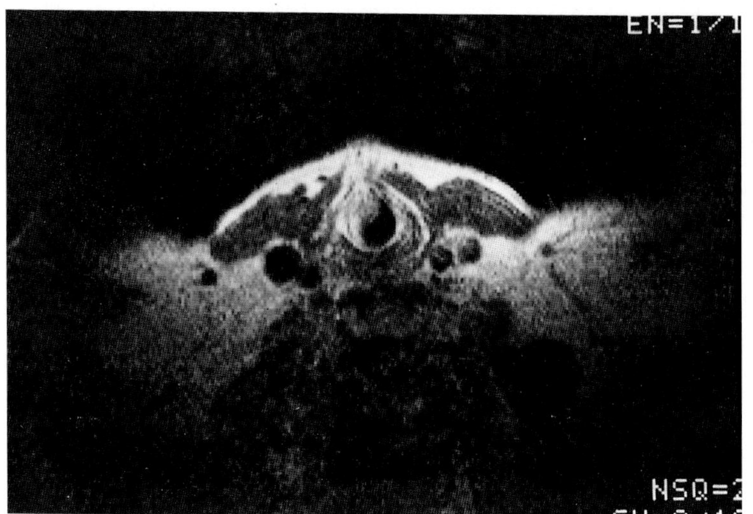

Fig. 13.6 Carcinoma of the larynx with subglottic extension and cartilage invasion (T4). *This 61-year-old man presented with hoarseness. A T2-weighted axial MRI examination (obtained using a shaped radiofrequency coil) at the level of the cricoid cartilage shows a subglottic mass encroaching on the airway. The tumor extends posteriorly and has invaded the cricoid cartilage. Because flowing blood does not generate a signal, the carotid artery and jugular vein appear as empty rings on MRI images. (Courtesy of A. Mancuso MD, Gainesville, Florida.)*

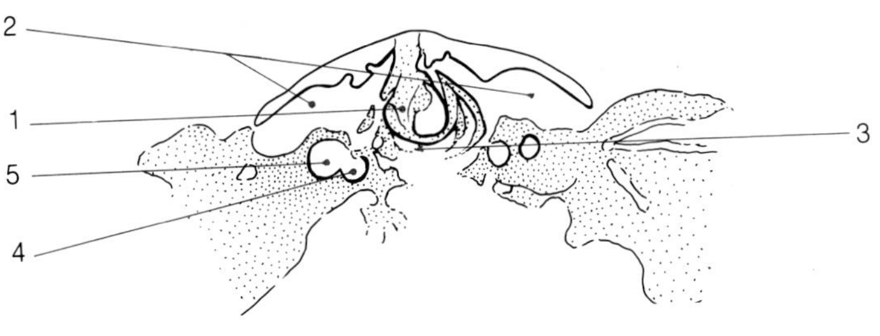

1 Tumor
2 Muscle
3 Invasion of cricoid cartilage
4 Carotid artery
5 Jugular vein

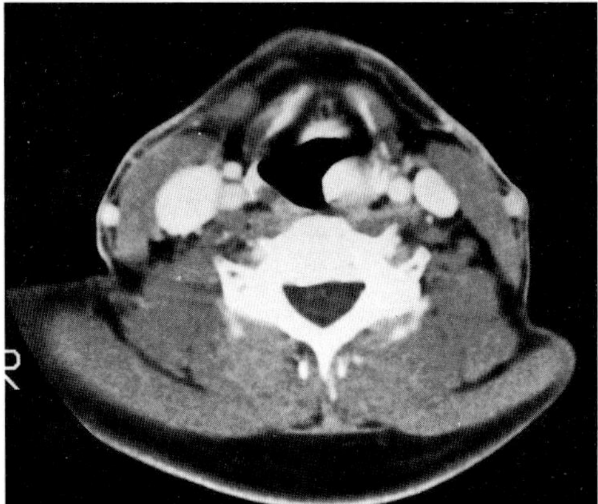

Fig. 13.7 Arteriovenous malformation of the aryepiglottic fold. *An axial contrast-enhanced CT scan in a 48-year-old man demonstrates an enhancing vascular mass in the left aryepiglottic fold. The mass enhances to the same degree as the ipsilateral common carotid artery and internal jugular vein.*

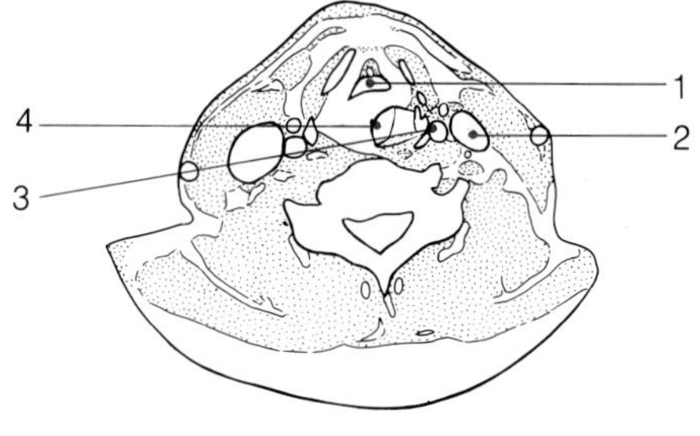

1 Epiglottis
2 Internal jugular vein
3 Common carotid artery
4 Enhancing vascular mass

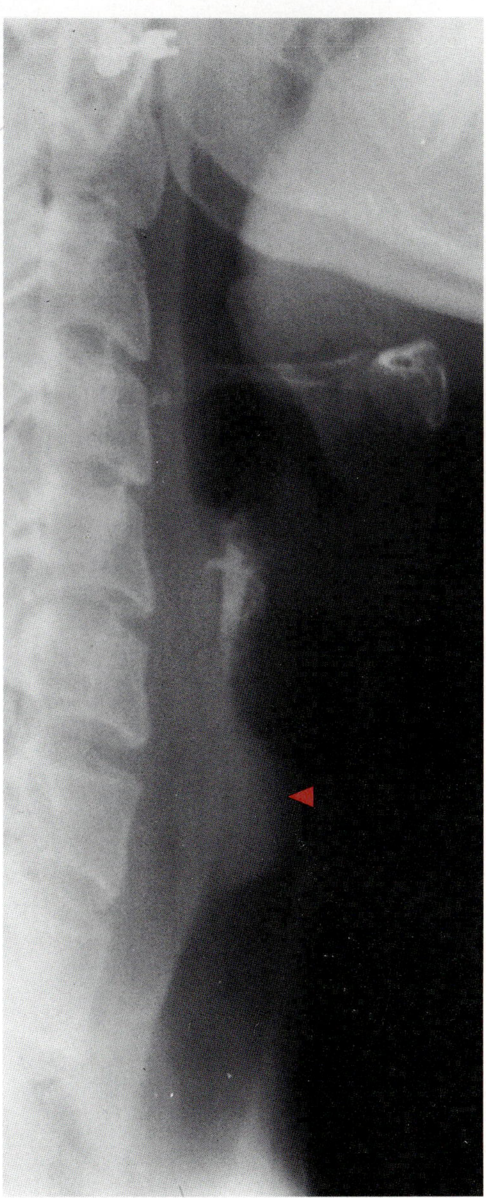

Fig. 13.8 Adenoid cystic carcinoma of the trachea. *A soft-tissue lateral radiograph of a 22-year-old woman shows a dome-shaped soft-tissue mass* (arrow) *encroaching on the tracheal airway. (Reproduced with permission from Noyek et al, 1985.)*

Upper Digestive Tract

The upper digestive tract comprises the oral cavity, pharynx, hypopharynx, and cervical esophagus.

ORAL CAVITY AND PHARYNX

Diagnostic imaging is not of primary importance in the assessment of soft-tissue lesions of the oral cavity, most of which are clinically accessible. However, imaging studies are important in the management of certain tumors and inflammatory disorders in which deep extension of disease is anticipated (see Chapter 8). Imaging techniques are also useful for lesions of the base of the tongue, which are often difficult to evaluate clinically.

Midline masses arising at the base of the tongue may be developmental or neoplastic in origin. The most common developmental mass is a lingual thyroid gland. On physical examination a lingual thyroid appears as a midline mass in the vicinity of the foramen cecum that elevates the overlying mucosa smoothly; typically the overlying mucosa appears somewhat hypervascular. The radioiodine scan is diagnostic and, perhaps more important, indicates whether there is functioning thyroid tissue present in its normal anatomic position (Fig. 14.1).

Infiltrating deep carcinomas of the base of the tongue are often occult, and cervical adenopathy may be the first clinical manifestation. In general, the primary tumor can be detected by CT or MRI before it is evident clinically (Fig. 14.2). Either modality can be used to monitor the response to treatment. Dynamic CT scanning will differentiate a cavernous hemangioma of the tongue from a malignant neoplasm, which it can mimic clinically (Fig. 14.3).

Retropharyngeal abscesses can usually be diagnosed on a lateral radiograph (Figs. 14.4). A barium swallow is sometimes needed to confirm the diagnosis in children, in whom physiologic variation in the thickness of the retrotracheal space can be a source of confusion. Opaque foreign objects that lodge in the hypopharynx or cervical esophagus are readily identified on plain films (Fig. 14.5). A fishbone or other radiolucent object can be demonstrated by having the patient swallow a barium-impregnated cotton pledget.

HYPOPHARYNX AND CERVICAL ESOPHAGUS

Structural and functional abnormalities of the hypopharynx and cervical esophagus (e.g., intrinsic and extrinsic masses, strictures, Zenker's diverticulum, impaired cricopharyngeal mobility) can be demonstrated by a fluoroscopically monitored barium swallow (Figs. 14.6, 14.7). Disorders of the swallowing mechanism (e.g., palatine incompetence, nasal reflux, laryngeal aspiration) are not uncommon in patients with neurologic disorders, and are best studied with rapid sequence of films or videotape recording. Extrinsic masses affecting the cervical esophagus are best evaluated by means of CT or MRI.

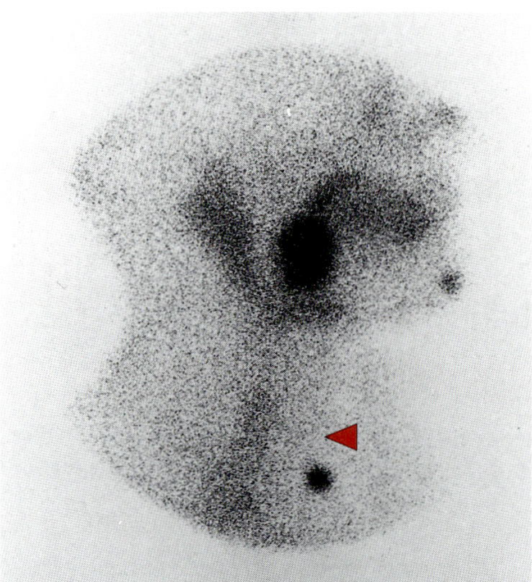

Fig. 14.1 Lingual thyroid gland. *This 31-year-old man presented with an asymptomatic mass at the base of the tongue, detected on routine mirror laryngoscopy. A lateral view of a pertechnetate scan shows focal accumulation of the radionuclide at the base of the tongue, indicating lingual thyroid gland. There is no uptake of the radionuclide in the usual anatomic position of the thyroid gland (arrow). The area of uptake in the neck is a suprasternal marker.*

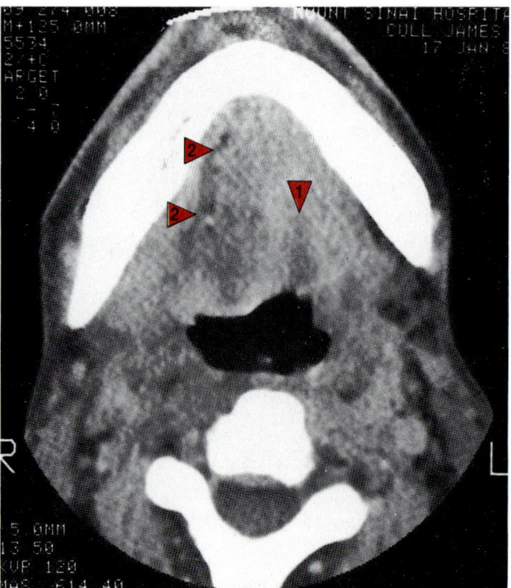

Fig. 14.2 Occult carcinoma of the base of the tongue. *This 48-year-old man presented with unilateral otalgia. Axial CT scan through the base of the tongue shows an ill-defined mass (arrow 1) in the left side of the tongue, which obliterates the normal fat planes; compare normal fat planes on right (arrows 2). The tumor crosses the midline.*

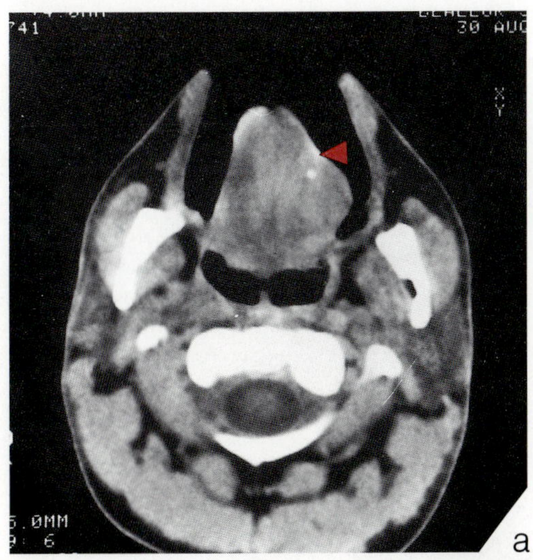

Fig. 14.3 Cavernous hemangioma of the tongue. *This 22-year-old man had noted a mass in the left half of his tongue for many years.* ***a*** *An axial CT scan (without contrast enhancement) demonstrates a bulky mass in the left half of the tongue. The presence of a calcified phlebolith (arrow) within the mass strongly suggests that it is a cavernous hemangioma.* ***b*** *A dynamic CT scan demonstrates the vascular pooling of contrast within the hemangioma in region 1 (compare with normal vascularity of the uninvolved right half of the tongue in region 2).*

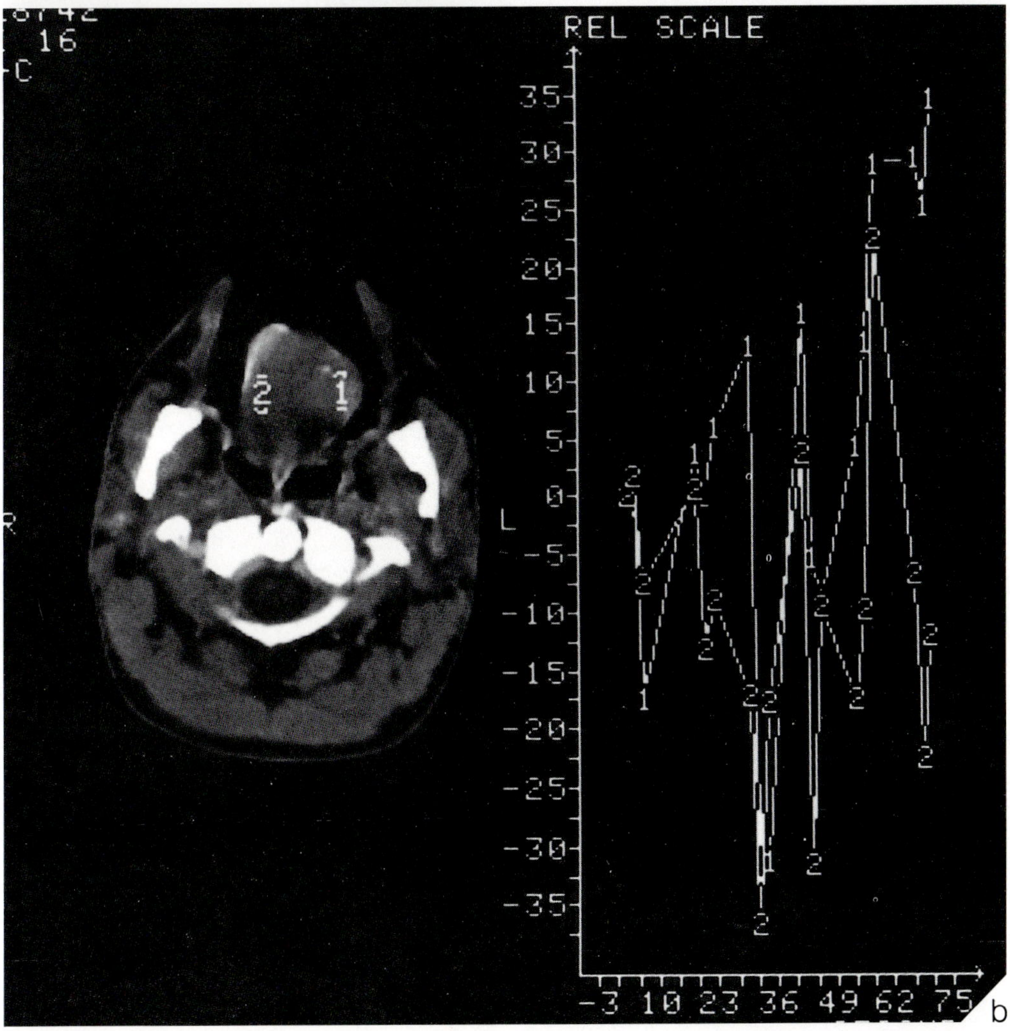

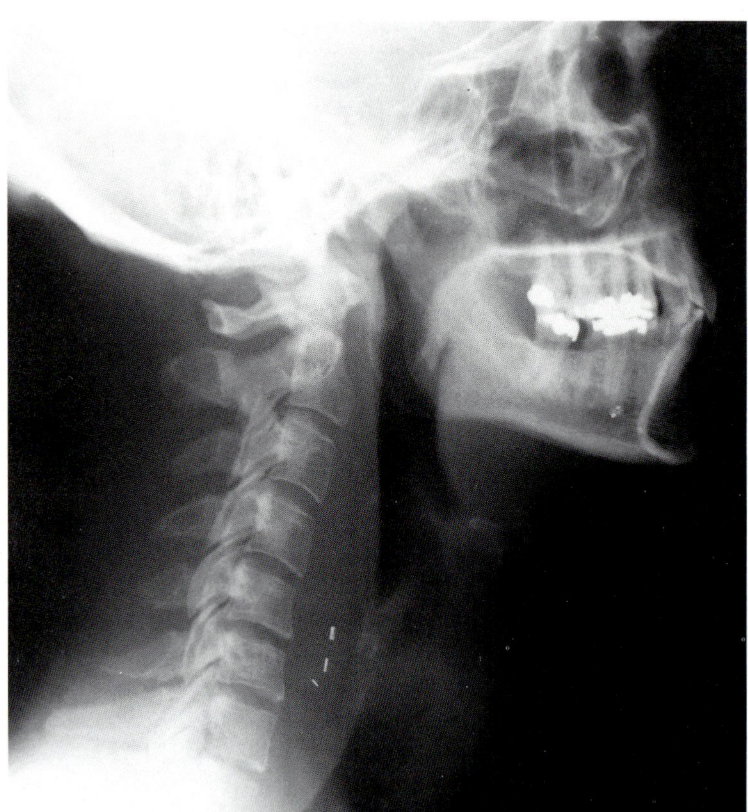

Fig. 14.4 Retropharyngeal abscess. *This 53-year-old man developed a retropharyngeal infection following a dental extraction. A lateral radiograph shows diffuse widening of the retropharyngeal space. (The thickness of the retropharyngeal soft tissues should not exceed the height of the adjacent vertebral body.) The swelling extends from the skull base to the thoracic inlet, and therefore involves the retroesophageal soft tissues as well.*

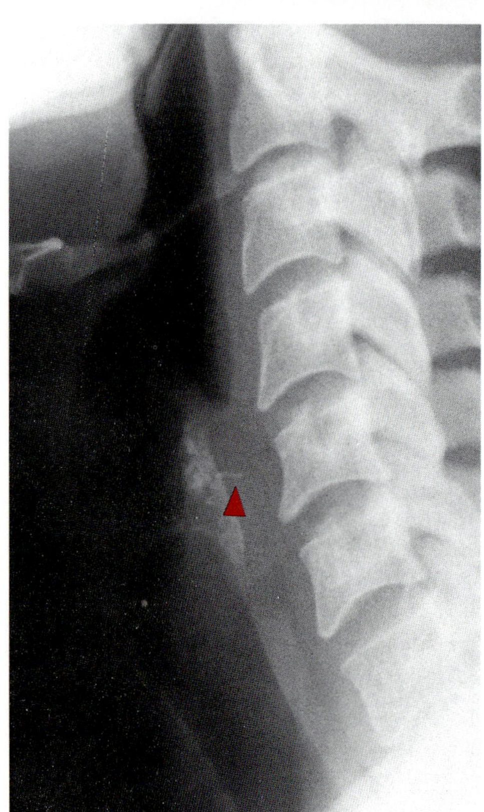

Fig. 14.5 Foreign body in the hypopharynx. *While eating a salad this 36-year-old woman "swallowed something that stuck in [her] throat." A lateral radiograph shows a small metal fragment (arrow) superimposed over the ala of the left thyroid cartilage. (The horizontal orientation of the foreign body clearly differentiates it from the adjacent thyroid cartilage, in which the calcification is vertically oriented.) At endoscopy, the metal fragment was found in the left piriform sinus.*

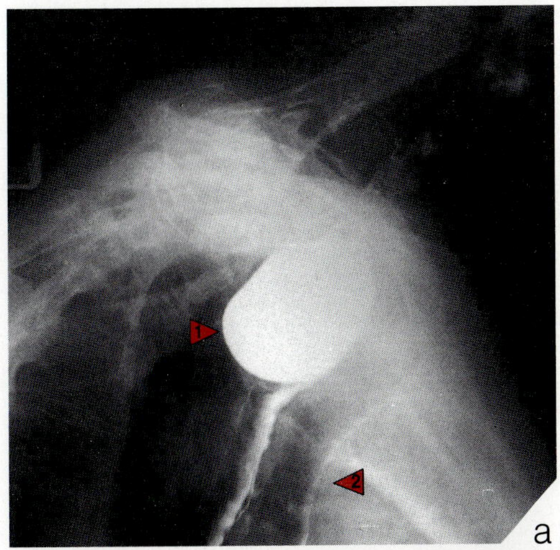

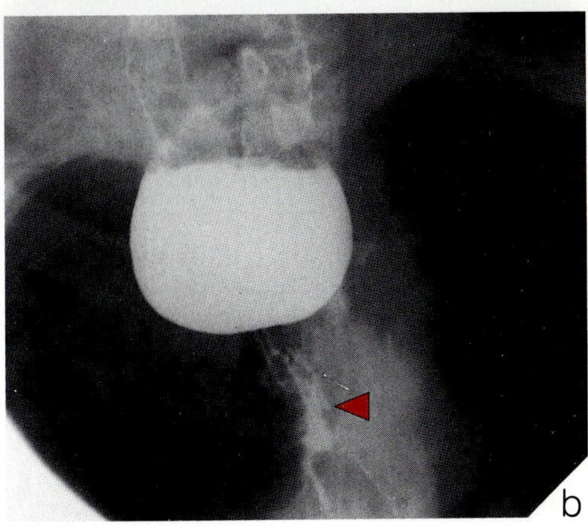

Fig. 14.6 Zenker's diverticulum of the hypopharynx. *An 84-year-old man with dysphagia.* **a** *An oblique projection of a barium swallow demonstrates a large esophageal diverticulum (arrow 1) arising in the neck and extending into the superior mediastinum. The diverticulum originates proximal to the cricopharyngeal sphincter (i.e., in the hypopharynx), and passes behind the esophagus to enter the mediastinum. The patient has aspirated a small amount of barium, which outlines the trachea (arrow 2).* **b** *A frontal erect spot film of the thoracic inlet shows an air–fluid level in the diverticulum. During fluoroscopy most of the barium entered the Zenker's diverticulum and only a small amount trickled into the thoracic esophagus (arrow).*

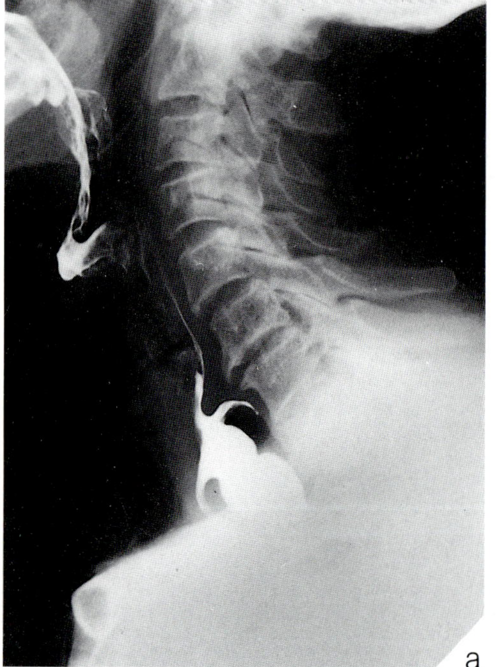
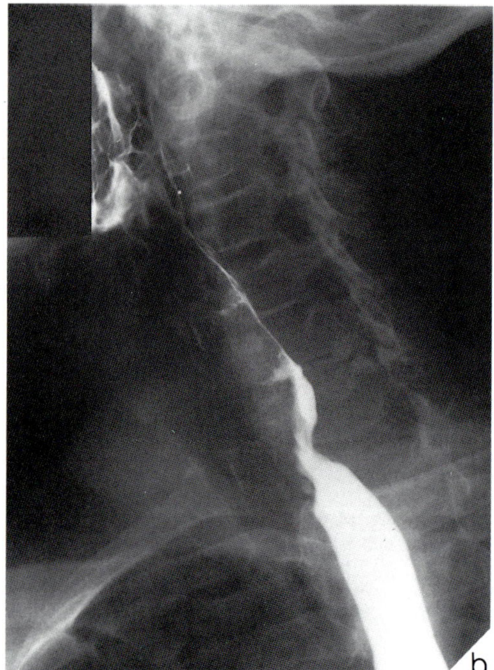

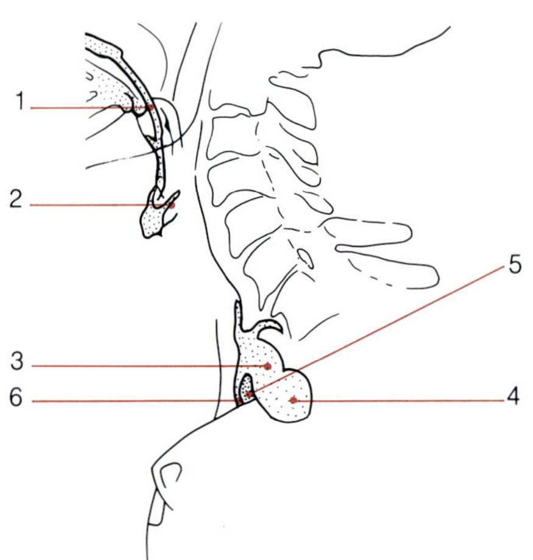

Fig. 14.7 Zenker's diverticulum of the hypopharynx. *A 77-year-old man with dysphagia.* ***a*** *Lateral view of an esophagram shows the characteristic anatomic relationships of a Zenker's diverticulum. The mouth of the diverticulum is just above the cricopharyngeus muscle sphincter at the junction of hypopharynx and cervical esophagus. The cervical esophagus is anterior to the cricopharyngeus, and anterior and below the mouth of the diverticulum.* ***b*** *A repeat esophagram 3 weeks following surgery shows normal flow of barium into the esophagus. The diverticulum is no longer seen.*

Vascular Lesions of the Head and Neck

In the past few years intraarterial embolization has been employed in many centers as the primary treatment for a variety of vascular lesions (e.g., paragangliomas, cavernous hemangiomas, arteriovenous malformations) of the head and neck, as well as to control intractable epistaxis. The larger vascular tumors (over 1 cm in diameter), as well as arteriovenous fistulas and intrinsic or extrinsic vascular obstructions, can be detected by intravenous DSA (Fig. 15.1), or by conventional arteriography (Fig. 15.2). Superselective catheter techniques may be needed to demonstrate very small lesions. Dynamic CT scanning provides further insight into the pathophysiology of these lesions (see Fig. 15.2a), and is helpful in planning the therapeutic approach. Before carrying out the embolization procedure, the arterial supply, morphology, and venous drainage of the lesion must be accurately mapped by superselective angiography (see Fig. 1.13).

Nonchromattin paragangliomas of the head and neck (e.g., carotid body tumors) may be multiple and familial. Therefore any patient with such a tumor (or a positive family history) should have a screening DSA to exclude additional tumors within the carotid distribution (see Fig. 15.1).

Cavernous hemangiomas have a predilection for certain locations (the parotid gland and its environs, the paranasal sinuses, and the larynx). A scintigraphic method, which employs the patient's own tagged red blood cells, has proved to be a simple and effective means of detecting these lesions (see Fig. 9.9).

A venous aneurysm is an unusual cause of a neck mass in a child or teenager. The diagnosis can be confirmed by Doppler ultrasound or venography (Fig. 15.3).

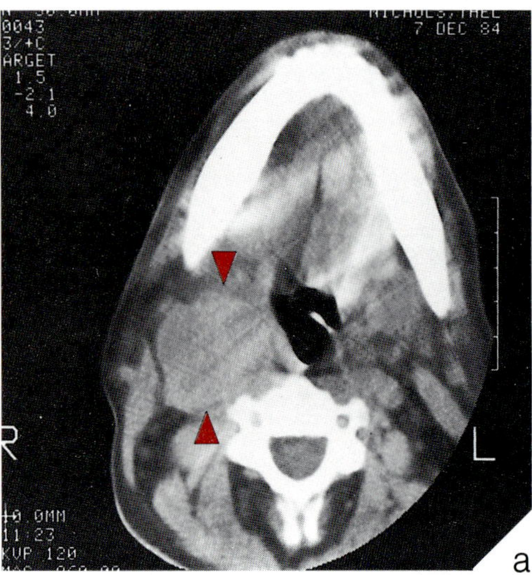

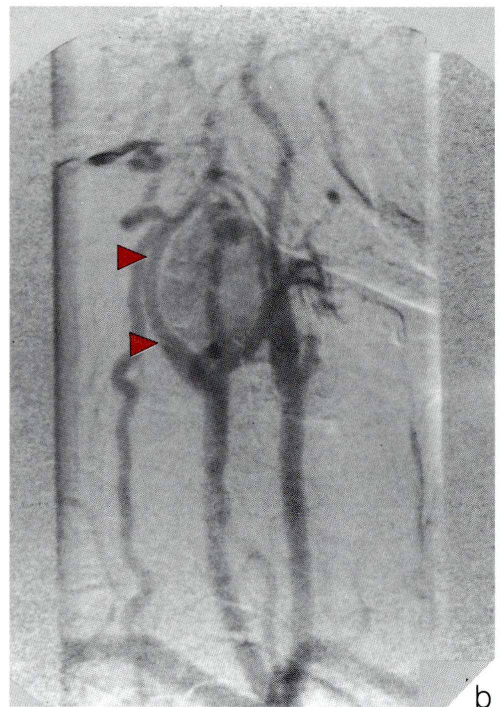

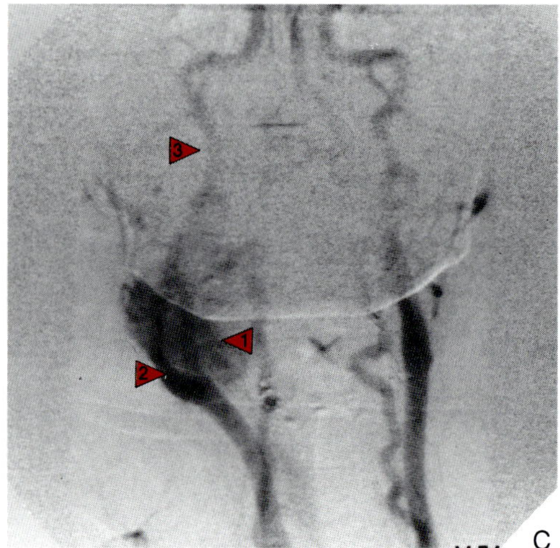

Fig. 15.1 Carotid body tumor. *This 53-year-old woman presented with a pulsatile neck mass.* ***a*** *Axial cut of CT scan at the level of the nasopharynx demonstrates an enhancing tumor mass (carotid body tumor) in the right parapharyngeal space. The tumor (arrows) encroaches on the nasopharyngeal air space and extends laterally into the neck (compare with the opposite side, where the normal fascial planes of the deep neck spaces are easily identified by their fat density).* ***b*** *Right oblique projection of a DSA (aortic arch injection) shows the typical vascular blush (arrows) of a carotid body tumor, which is supplied by branches of the carotid artery. The tumor displaces the internal and external carotid arteries at the bifurcation.* ***c*** *The anteroposterior projection view further defines the relationships of the tumor. The vascular tumor (arrow 1) lies in the crotch between the internal and external carotid arteries. The proximal portion of the internal carotid artery (arrow 2) is bowed laterally around the mass; beyond the mass the course of the internal carotid artery is normal (arrow 3). (Note: Since nonchromattin paragangliomas can be multiple, the entire cephalic distribution of the aortic arch must be visualized to exclude additional tumors.)*

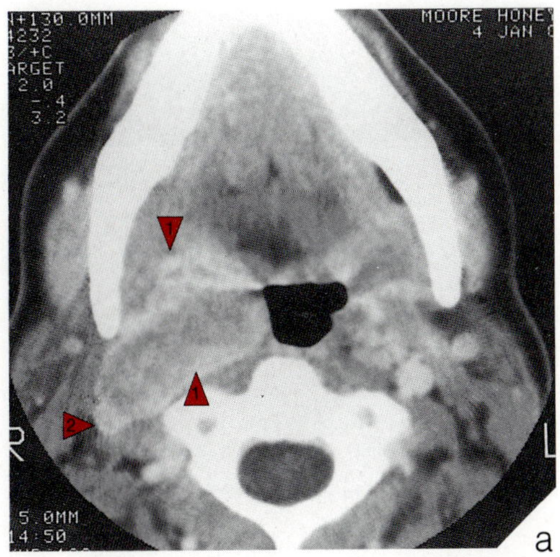

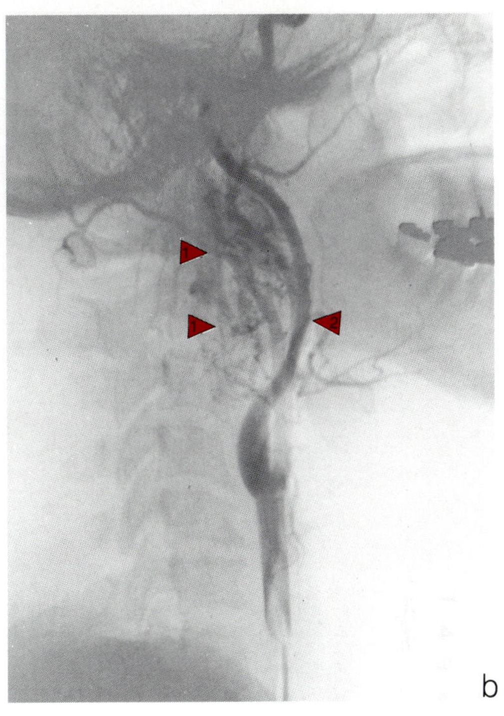

Fig. 15.2 Glomus vagale tumor. *a* *A contrast-enhanced axial CT scan demonstrates a large mass, a glomus vagale tumor (arrows 1), in the right parapharyngeal space. The periphery of the mass enhances but the central portion is relatively hypodense. The mass encroaches on the nasopharynx and extends into the deep fascial spaces of the neck, displacing the internal carotid artery laterally (arrow 2).* ***b*** *A lateral projection of a conventional carotid arteriogram shows a tangle of small vessels (arrows 1) supplied by branches of the external carotid artery. The vascular tumor abuts the internal carotid artery, which is bowed anteriorly (arrow 2).*

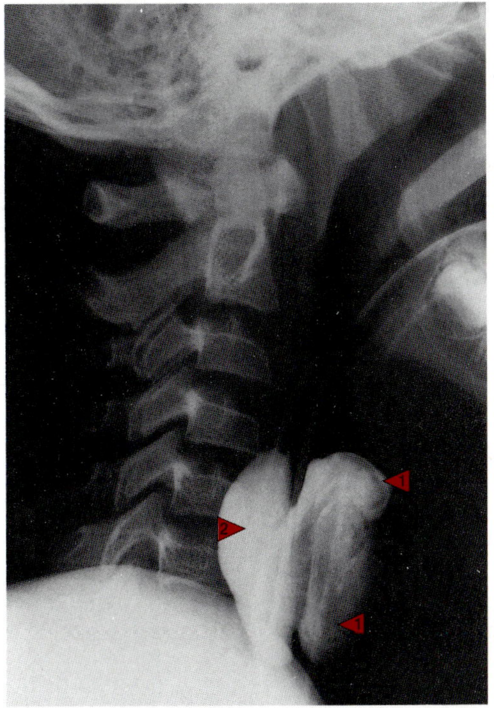

Fig. 15.3 Spontaneous aneurysm of the internal jugular vein (jugular venous estasia). *This 11-year-old boy presented with a slowly enlarging mass in the anterolateral aspect of the neck. A lateral view of a direct jugular venogram shows a large aneurysm (arrows 1) projecting anteriorly from the internal jugular vein (arrow 2). There was no history of trauma, sepsis, hypertension, congenital heart disease, or connective tissue disorder, and this presumably represents a "spontaneous" aneurysm. (Courtesy of J. Friedberg, MD, Toronto, Canada.)*

Nonvascular Soft-Tissue Lesions of the Neck

Soft-tissue masses of the neck are classified as midline or lateral; a variety of cystic and solid lesions occur at each location. Thyroglossal duct cysts and thyroglossal duct remnants are the most frequently encountered midline masses. Dermoids also occur in the midline but are much less common. Nonvascular masses occurring in the lateral neck include branchial cleft cysts; enlarged lymph nodes due to inflammation, metastasis, or nonspecific hypertrophy; lipomas; cystic hygromas (lymphangiomas); and neurogenic tumors (e.g., schwannomas).

While a careful clinical examination usually suffices in most patients with midline or lateral neck masses, sonography can be helpful if the diagnosis is in doubt (Fig. 16.1). A branchial cleft cyst typically appears as a discrete cystic structure situated at the junction of the upper and middle thirds of the stemomastoid muscle, deep to the posterior border of the muscle. It is sometimes very difficult to differentiate a branchial cleft cyst from a necrotic lymph node by sonography. Draining tracts in the lateral neck generally represent branchial cleft fistulas. By injecting contrast media into the tract (fistulography), it is often possible to demonstrate communication with the pharynx or other deep structures.

Lipomas are characterized by their fat density on CT (Fig. 16.2) and their highly echogenic appearance on sonography. While a well-encapsulated lipoma is easily diagnosed by clinical examination, diffuse fatty infiltration of the soft tissues may be difficult to distinguish from a cystic hygroma. A sonogram will resolve any doubts.

Neurogenic tumors (schwannomas) occasionally occur in the lateral neck. On palpation these tumors move in lateral direction only, which may suggest the diagnosis to an astute clinician. Neurogenic tumors have a characteristic appearance on CT (Fig. 16.3).

CT of the neck is indispensable in the pretreatment staging of head and neck cancer. It also plays a crucial role in the management of patients with cervical node metastases in whom a thorough investigation of the upper aerodigestive tract, including sophisticated telescopic examinations, has failed to uncover a primary malignant focus. Often the occult primary is a microscopic lesion in the nasopharynx, base of tongue, or tonsillar region. A meticulous CT examination—which should include the entire neck from the skull base to the thoracic inlet—will not only document the number and distribution of abnormal lymph nodes, but may identify an occult primary as well. CT is especially helpful in heavy-set patients in whom clinical assessment of cervical nodes is difficult.

Lymph nodes appear as discrete, nonenhancing structures on the CT scan (Figs. 16.4, 16.5). Dynamic CT scans can help differentiate small lymph nodes from arteries, which is sometimes difficult on a conventional scan. Necrotic lymph nodes are presumed to be malignant in patients with a known primary (see Figs. 16.4, 16.5). While size is not an absolute criterion of malignancy, larger lymph nodes are more likely to harbor metastases than smaller ones. Nodes in the 1.5 to 2.0 cm range may or may not be pathologic; nodes measuring 2.0 to 2.5 cm should be regarded with suspicion; and nodes measuring 2.5 cm and larger are usually malignant. Lymphomatous lymph nodes are typically homogeneous and echo-poor, and can be mistaken for cysts on sonography.

MRI promises to be an important advance in the investigation of cervical adenopathy. One inherent advantage of MRI over CT is that blood vessels—which are devoid of signal— are easily differentiated from lymph nodes. Whether MRI can consistently differentiate malignant from nonmalignant nodes is still uncertain.

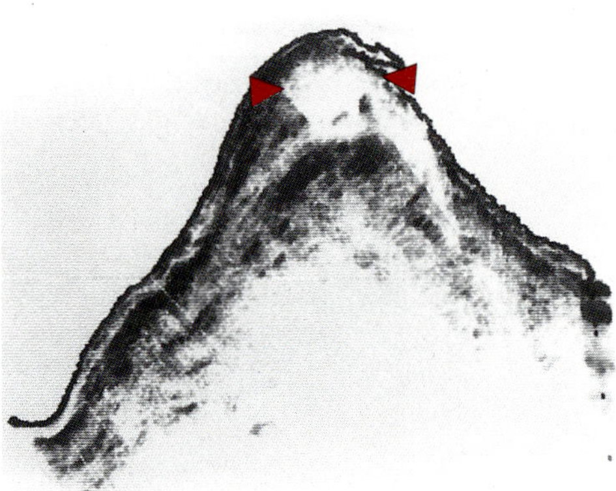

Fig. 16.1 Thyroglossal duct cyst. *A high-resolution axial sonogram in a 33-year-old woman who presented with a painless midline suprahyoid mass, shows a 1.5 cm cystic structure* (arrows) *with excellent through transmission.*

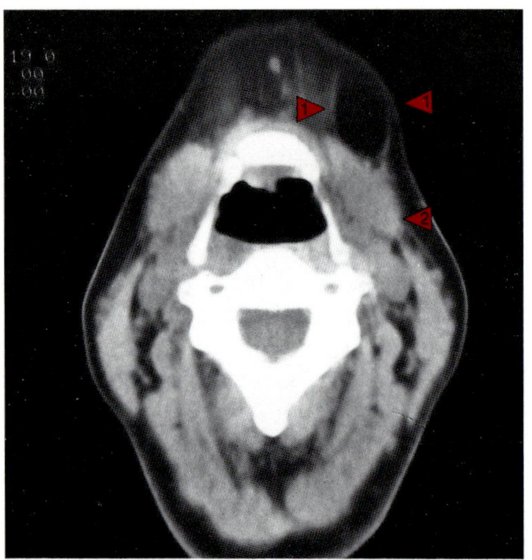

Fig. 16.2 Lipoma of the left submandibular region. *An axial CT scan shows a well circumscribed low attenuation lesion, lipoma (arrows 1), below and anterior to the left submandibular gland (arrow 2), which is not involved. The lesion has the same CT number as the adjacent subcutaneous fat.*

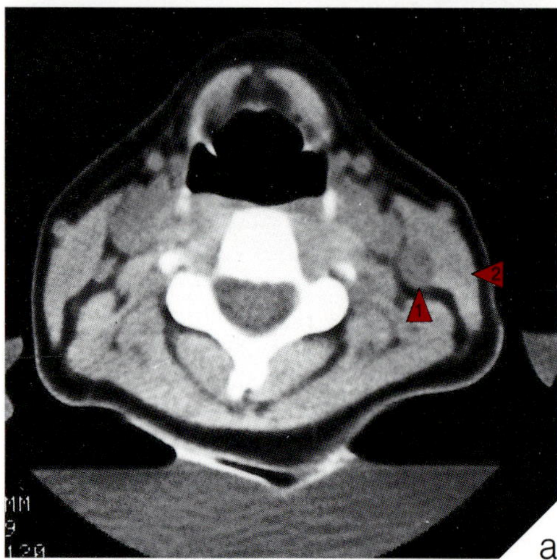

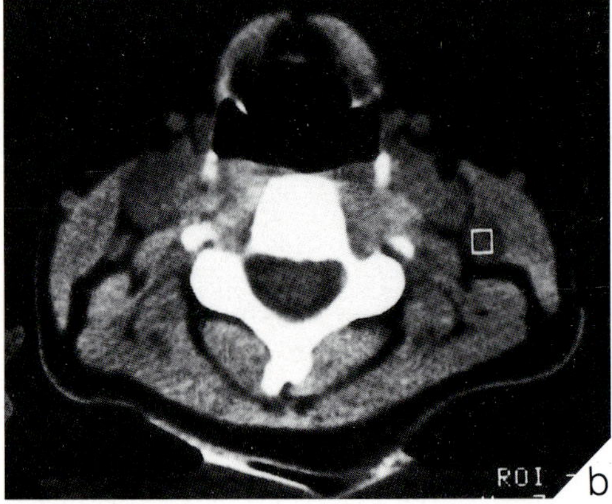

Fig. 16.3 Schwannoma of the spinal accessory nerve. *a An axial CT scan shows a small low-attenuation mass (arrow 1) impressing the posterior surface of the sternomastoid muscle (arrow 2). b Same cut photographed with narrow window shows the lesion to advantage. The CT number (region under cursor) is 43 Hounsfield units, consistent with nerve tissue. (Reproduced with permission from McShane et al, 1986.)*

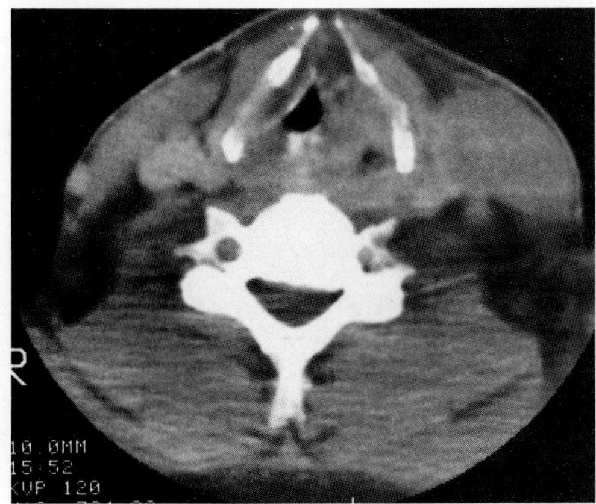

Fig. 16.4 Carcinoma of the left piriform sinus with cervical lymph node metastases. *An axial contrast-enhanced CT scan in a 45-year-old man with squamous cell carcinoma of the left piriform sinus shows two large, centrally necrotic lymph nodes, with minimal but definite peripheral vascular enhancement. The left piriform sinus is filled with necrotic tumor (note central ulceration).*

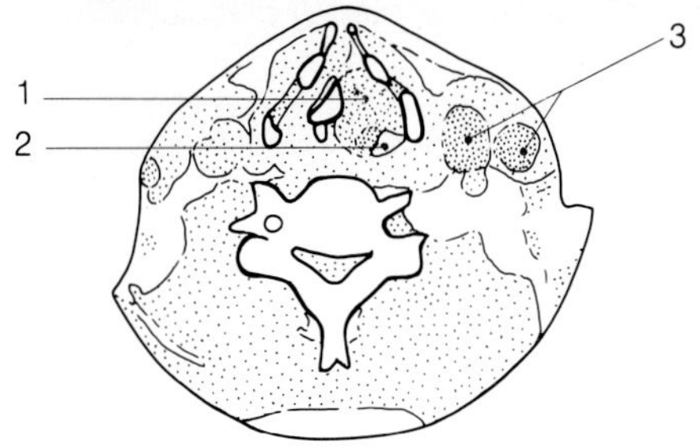

Fig. 16.5 Papillary carcinoma of the thyroid gland with "cystic" lymph node metastasis.
This 29-year-old man presented with a large, soft deep-cervical mass in the left lower neck.
a *A pertechnetate thyroid scan (anterior view) demonstrates a "cold" nodule (arrow 1) in the upper portion of the left thyroid lobe.* ***b*** *An axial CT scan at the level of the thyroid shows a large mass on the left (under cursor), which represents a lymph node metastasis. Because of the its low CT number (32 Hounsfield units), the mass was initially thought to represent a branchial cleft cyst.* ***c*** *A high-resolution transverse (axial) sonogram at the level of the thyroid gland shows a large hypoechoic structure just to the left of the carotid artery. The absence of internal echos, prominent backwall reverberation artifact, and good through transmission are typical of a fluid-containing structure ("cyst"). However, there is a papillary projection of tumor into the "cyst," indicating that it is a necrotic lymph node metastasis. The left thyroid lobe is enlarged but no definite mass is seen.* ***d*** *A longitudinal (parasagittal) scan shows compression of the internal jugular vein (arrows 4) by the enlarged, hypoechoic lymph node. A small papillary projection of tumor (arrow 5) into the central portion of the predominantly cystic lymph node is also seen in this projection.*

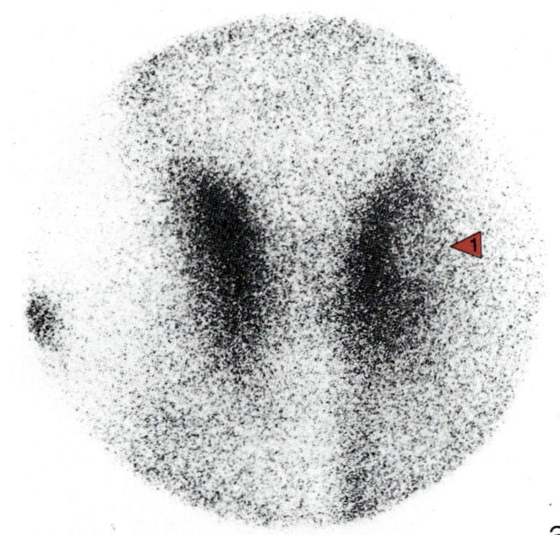

a

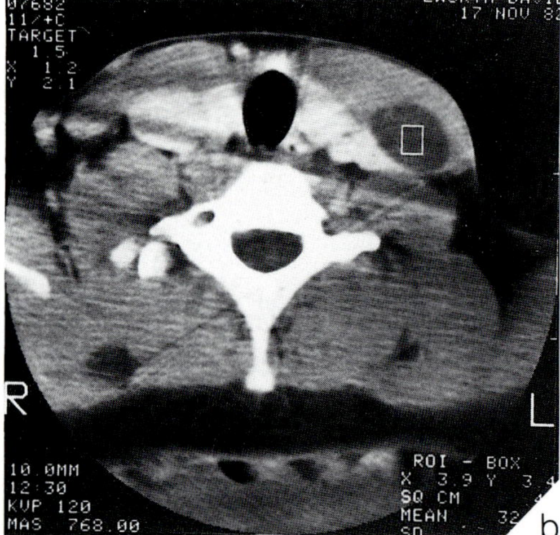

b

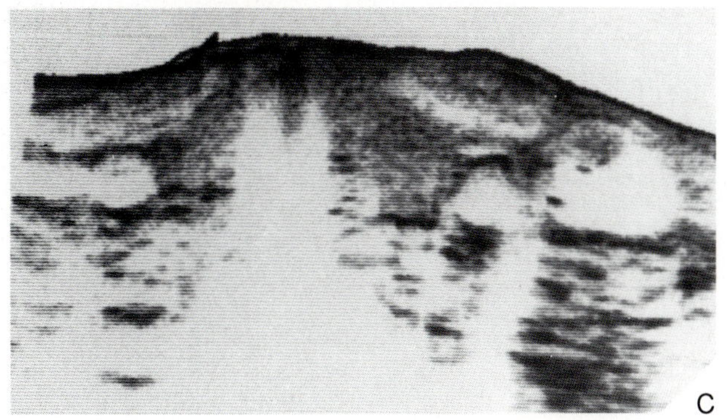

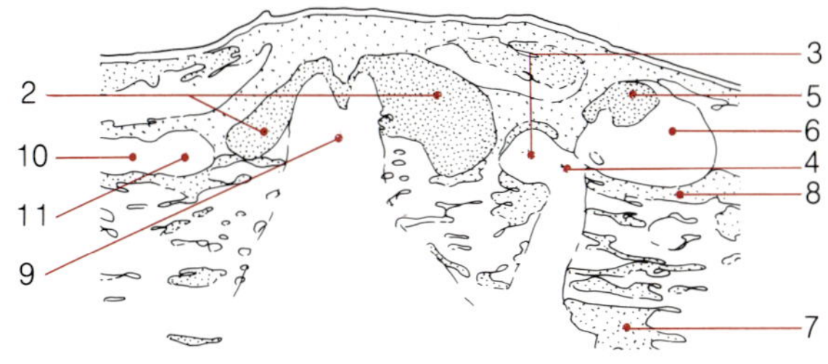

1 Cold nodule
2 Thyroid lobes
3 Left common carotid artery
4 Compressed left internal jugular vein
5 Papillary projection of tumor
6 Enlarged necrotic lymph node
7 Increased through transmission
8 Back wall reverberation artifact
9 Trachea
10 Right internal jugular vein
11 Right common carotid artery

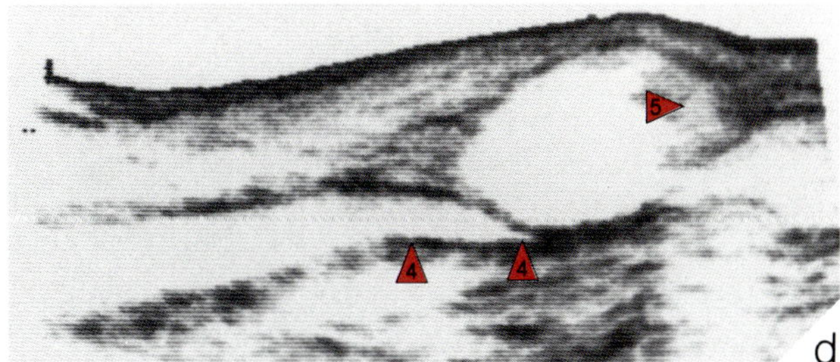

Otolaryngologic Manifestations of Systemic Disease

A great many systemic disorders can affect the soft tissues and bony structures of the head and neck, including infections (e.g., tuberculosis); vasculitides (e.g., Wegener's granulomatosis, systemic lupus erythematosis); metabolic disorders (Fig. 17.1); Paget's disease (Fig 17.2): neurofibromatosis (see Fig. 17.5) and a variety of neoplasms (Fig. 17.3); arthropathies (see Fig. 8.2); bone dysplasias (see Fig. 7.1); and congenital malformations. Many of the imaging techniques described in this chapter play a role in the management of these diverse conditions.

Fig. 17.1 Multiple brown tumors secondary to hyperparathyroidism. *A 55-year-old man with primary hyperparathyroidism secondary to parathyroid carcinoma.* ***a*** *A coronal tomogram of the left maxillary sinus demonstrates a soft-tissue density within the left maxillary sinus and above it. The roof of the maxillary sinus appears to be intact.* ***b*** *An oblique radiograph of the mandible shows a corticated mass (arrows 2) within the body of the mandible.* ***c*** *A lateral view of a technetium 99m diphosphonate bone scan (delayed phase) shows increased uptake (osteoblastic response) in the maxillary and mandibular lesions (arrows 4).* ***d*** *Posterior view of the thorax from the same bone scan shows uptake in brown tumors of the right fifth rib and right scapula (arrows 4).* ***e*** *Radiograph shows an expansile destructive lesion (arrows 5) of the right fifth rib. The radiographic findings are characteristic of a brown tumor. (Reproduced with permission from Noyek et al, 1977.)*

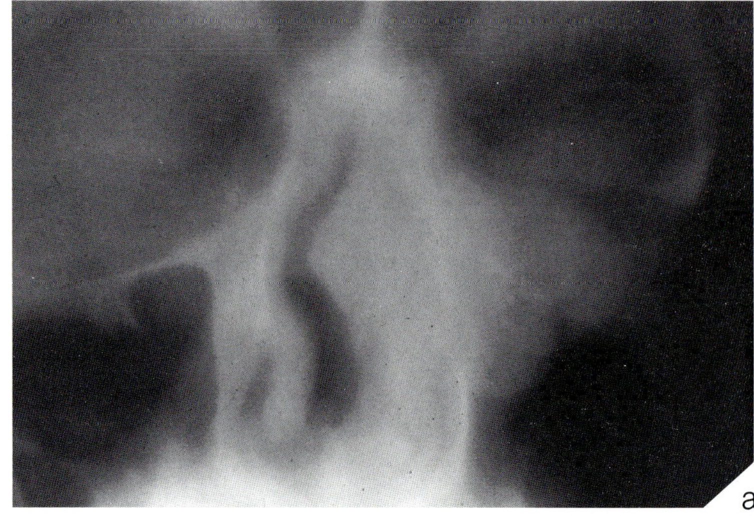

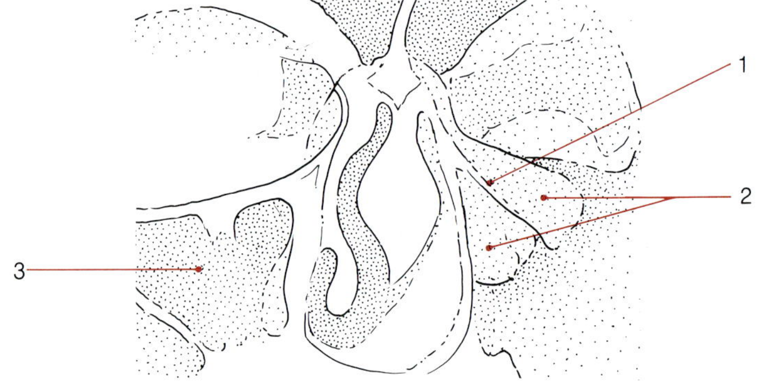

1 Roof of left maxillary sinus
2 Mass
3 Right maxillary sinus
4 Increased uptake
5 Decreased uptake

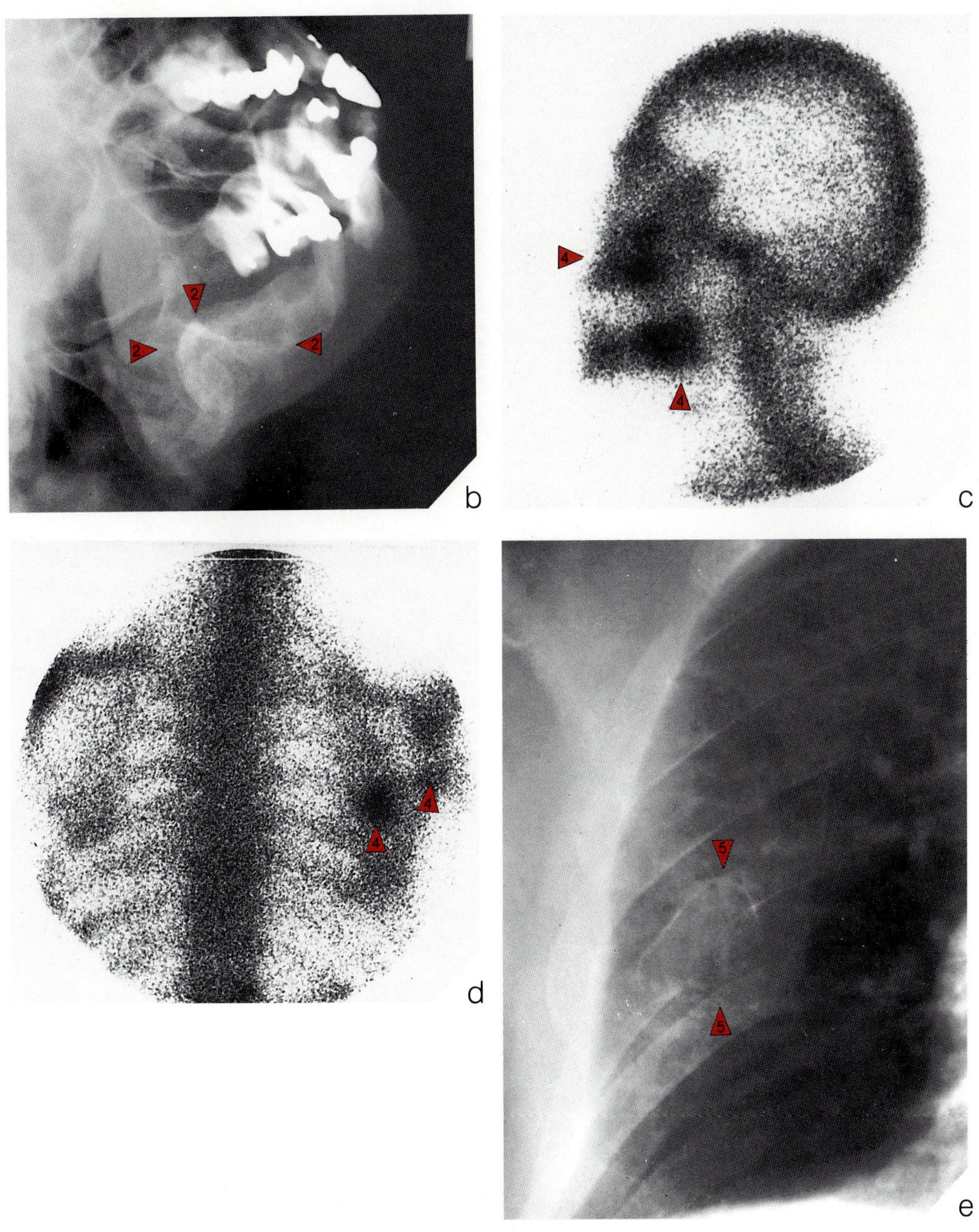

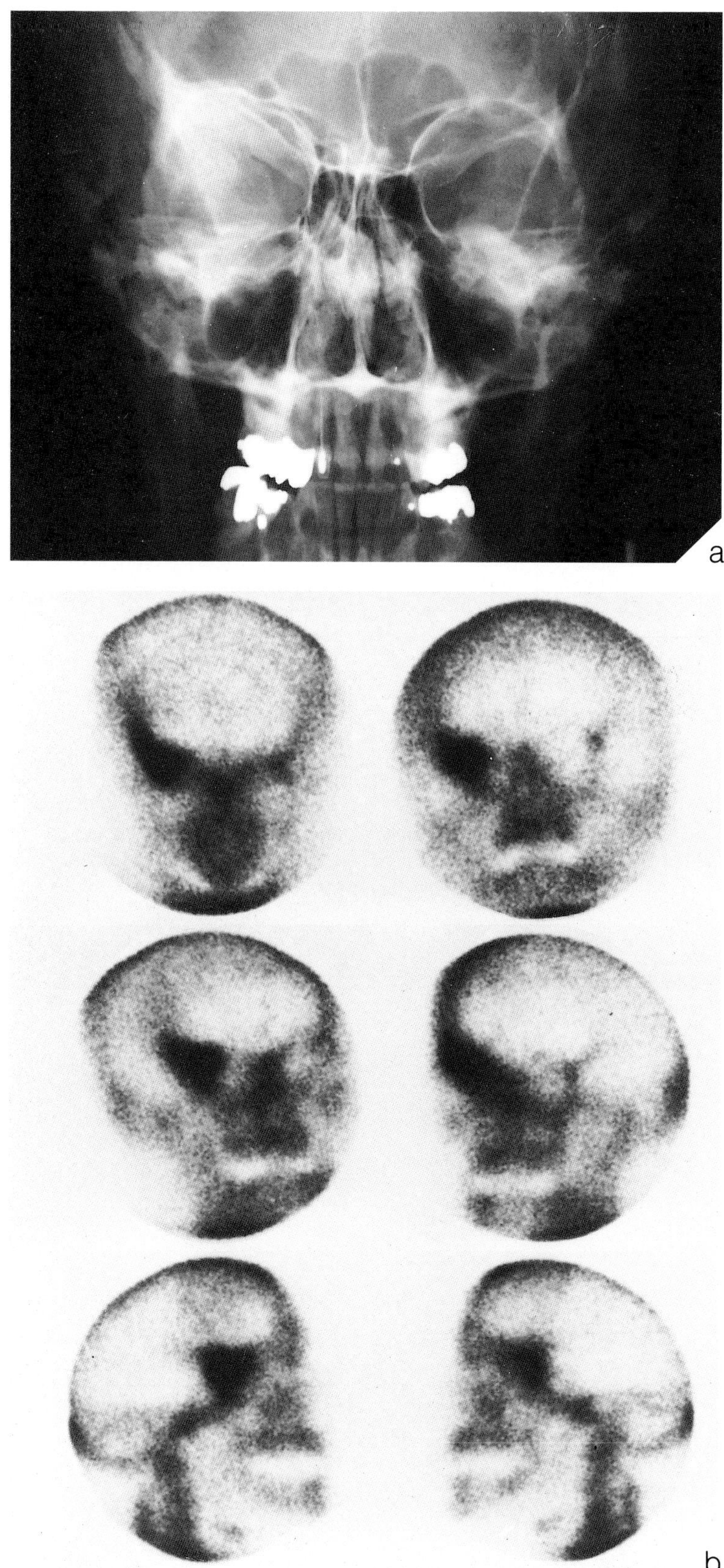

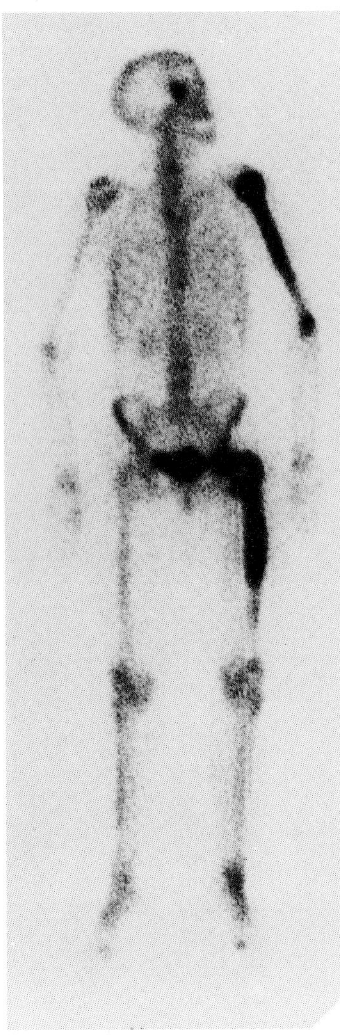

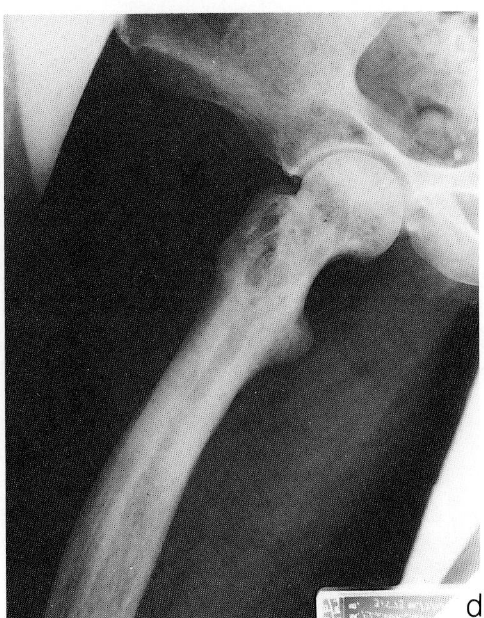

Fig. 17.2 Paget's disease involving the skull base. *a A Caldwell projection shows osteoblastic changes in both the greater and lesser wings of the right sphenoid bone (compare with normal structures on left). Although these findings are compatible with Paget's disease, meningioma would be the first diagnostic possibility.* ***b*** *Delayed phase of an MDP bone scan, in multiple projections (clockwise from upper left: Ant, Waters, LAO, LL, RL, RAO) shows increased uptake in the right sphenoid bone.* ***c*** *The whole-body bone scan (anterior view) shows increased uptake in the right humerus and proximal half of the right femur, indicating osteoblastic activity.* ***d*** *A plain film shows typical changes of Paget's disease in the head and shaft of the right femur. (Reproduced with permission from Noyek et al, 1979.)*

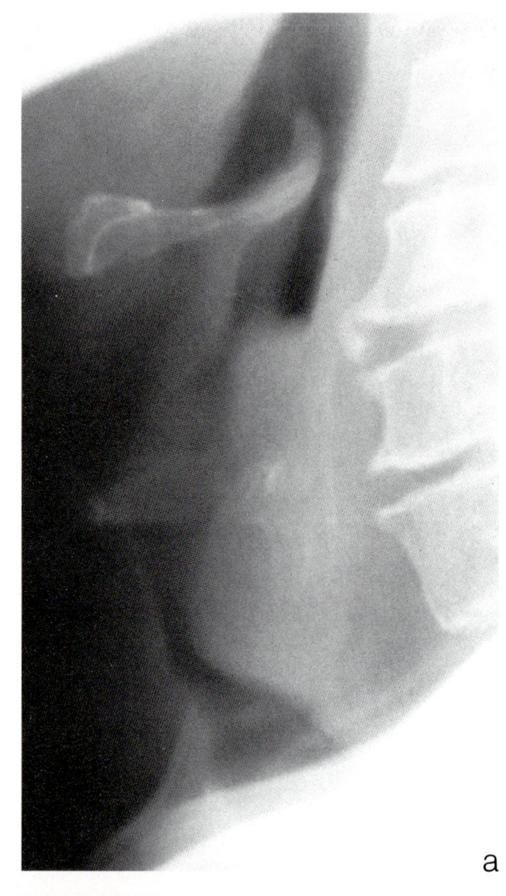

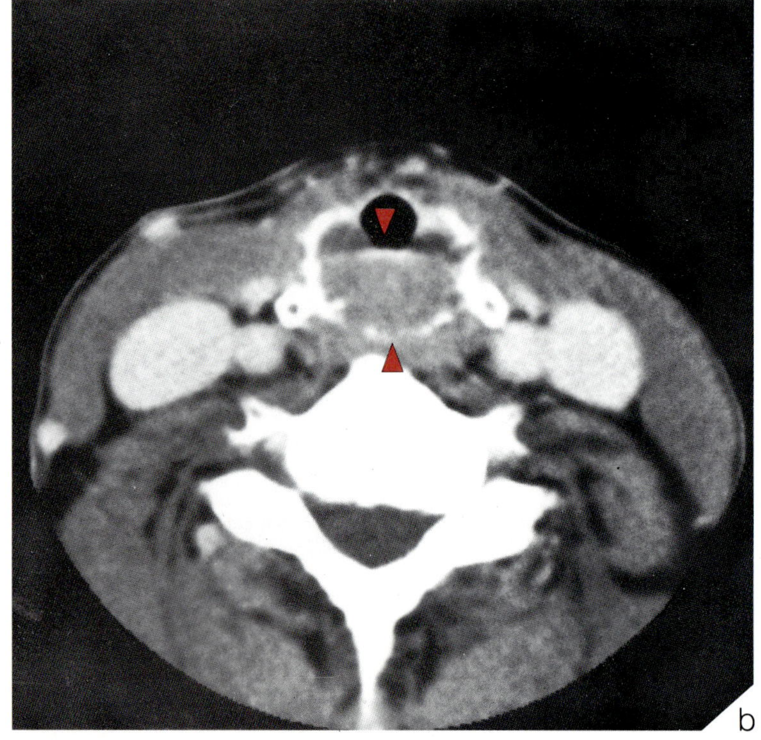

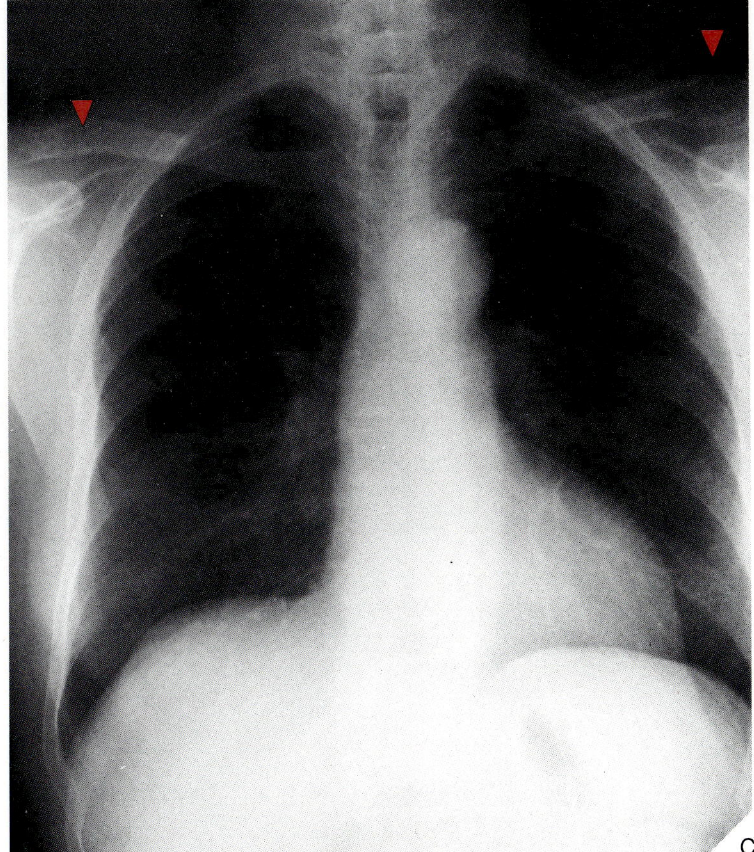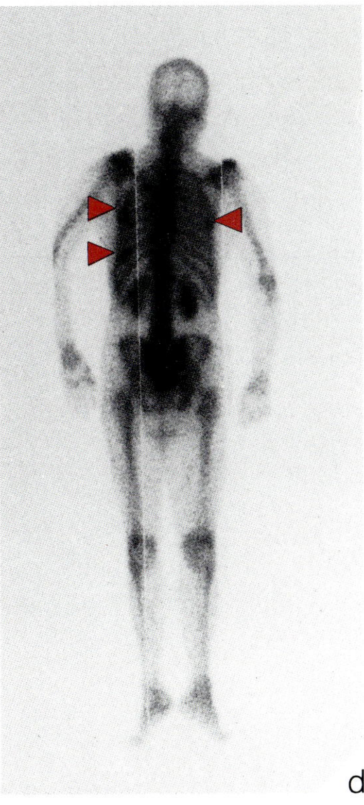

Fig. 17.3 Multiple myeloma involving the larynx.
*a A lateral radiograph shows a soft-tissue mass encroaching on the subglottic air space. **b** An axial CT scan shows expansion of the posterior lamina of the cricoid cartilage (arrows) by the tumor. **c** A chest radiograph shows typical destructive lesions of multiple myeloma (arrows) in the distal portion of each clavicle. **d** Posterior view of an MDP bone scan shows increased uptake in three ribs (arrows), indicating osteoblastic response to myeloma. (Reproduced with permission from Rutka J et al, 1985.)*

BIBLIOGRAPHY

Batsakis JG: Tumors of the Head and Neck: Clinical and Pathologic Considerations. Baltimore, Williams & Wilkins, 1979.

Bohman LL et al: CT approach to benign nasopharyngeal masses. AJNR 1:513, 1980.

Brandt-Zawadzki M et al: High-resolution CT with image reformation in maxillofacial pathology. ANJR 3:31,1982.

Daniels DL, Pech P, Haughton VM: Magnetic Resonance Imaging of the Temporal Bone. Milwaukee, General Electric Company Medical Systems Group, 1984.

Fitz CR, Noyek AM: Contemporary radiology in congenital craniofacial disorders. Otolaryngol Clin North Am 14:65, 1981.

Lufkin RB, Larsson SG, Hanafee WN: Work in progress: NMR anatomy of the larynx and tongue base. Radiology 148:173, 1983.

McShane D et al: Schwannoma of the intrasternomastoid portion of the spinal accessory nerve. J Otolaryngol 15:282, 1986.

Mafee MF et al: Computed tomography of the larynx: correlation with anatomic and pathologic studies in cases of laryngeal carcinoma. Radiology 147:123,1983.

Mancuso M, Hanafee WN: Elusive head and neck cancers beneath intact mucosa. Laryngoscope 93:133, 1983.

Mancuso M, Hanafee WN: Computed Tomography and Magnetic Resonance Imaging of the Head and Neck, 2nd edn. Baltimore, Williams & Wilkins, 1985.

Muraki AS, Mancuso M, Harnsberger HR: Metastatic cervical adenopathy from tumors of unknown origin: the role of CT. Radiology 152:749, 1984.

Noyek AM: Bone scanning in otolaryngology. Laryngoscope (suppl 18), 89:1, 1979.

Noyek AM et al: Xeroradiology in the assessment of the pediatric larynx and trachea. J Otolaryngol 5:469, 1976.

Noyek AM et al: Clinically-directed CT in occult disease of the skull base involving foramen ovale. Laryngoscope 91:1021,1982.

Noyek AM et al: Contemporary radiologic evaluation in maxillofacial trauma. Otolaryngol Clin North Am 16:473,1983.

Noyek AM et al: The clinical significance of radionuclide bone and gallium scanning in osteomyelitis of the head and neck. Laryngoscope (suppl 34), 94:1,1984.

Noyek AM et al: Radiologic evaluation of the larynx. In Bailey BJ, Biller HF (eds): Surgery of the Larynx. Philadelphia, Saunders, 1985.

Noyek AM, Greyson MD: Radionuclide scanning. In Blitzer A, Friedman WH, Lawson W (eds): Surgery of the Paranasal Sinuses. Philadelphia, Saunders, 1985.

Noyek AM, Wortzman G, Kassel EE: Diagnostic imaging in rhinology. In Goldman JL (ed.): Modern Rhinology. New York, John Wiley, 1987.

Osborn A, Hanafee WN, Mancuso AA: Normal and pathologic CT anatomy of the mandible. AJR 139:555, 1982.

Reede DL, Whelan MA, Bergeron RT: Computed tomography of the infrahyoid neck—parts 1 and 11. Radiology 145:389,1982.

Rothberg R et al: Thyroid cartilage imaging with diagnostic ultrasound. Arch Otolaryngol 112:503, 1986.

Rutka J et al: Multiple myeloma involving the cricoid cartilage. J Otolaryngol, 14:309, 1985.

Shaffer KA, Haughton VM, Wilson CR: High-resolution computed tomography of the temporal bone. Radiology 134:409,1980.

Som PM, Biller HF: The combined CT sialogram. Radiology 135:387, 1980.

Som PM et al: Computed tomography of glomus tympanicum tumors. J Comput Assist Tomogr 7:14, 1983.

Som PM, Shugar JM: Antral mucoceles: a new look. J Comput Assist Tomogr 4:484, 1980.

Som PM, Shugar JM, Biller HF: The early detection of antral malignancy in the postmaxillectomy patient. Radiology 143:509, 1982.

Zizmor J, Noyek AM: An Atlas of Otolaryngologic Radiology. Philadelphia, Saunders, 1978.

Zonneveld FW et al: Direct Multiplanar, High-Resolution, Thin Section of the Orbit. Eindhoven, The Netherlands, Philips Medical Systems Division, 1985.

INDEX

Note: The numbers in **boldface** refer to Figure numbers.

Abscess
extradural, with frontal sinusitis, 49, **6.1**
of parotid gland, 66, 69, **9.4**
retropharyngeal, 93, 96, **14.4**
Acoustic nerve, 1, 3, **1.1**
Acoustic neuroma, 2, 9, 10, **1.7–1.9**
bilateral, 3, 13, **1.12**
Adenoma
parathyroid, 79, 80, **11.1, 11.2**
thyroid, 73–75, 79, 80, **10.2, 10.3, 11.2**
parathyroid adenoma with, 79, 80, **11.2**
Air–fluid level
in maxillary sinus, 17, 21, **2.5**
in Zenker's diverticulum of hypopharynx, 93, 97, **14.6**
Aneurysm, jugular vein, 99, 101, **15.3**
Angiofibroma, nasopharyngeal, 19, 29, **2.16**
Angiography
in carotid body tumor, 99, 100, **15.1**
in glomus jugulare tumors, 3, 14, **1.13**
in glomus vagale tumor, 99, 101, **15.2**
in goiter extension into superior mediastinum, 81, 82, **12.1**
Aryepiglottic fold, arteriovenous malformation of, 85, 90, **13.7**
Auditory canal
external, 1, 3, **1.1**
congenital bony atresia of, 2, 8, **1.6**
fracture of floor, 2, 7, **1.5**
internal, 1, 3, **1.1**

Brown tumor in hyperparathyroidism, 109, 110, **17.1**

Calcium pyrophosphate dihydrate deposition disease of temporomandibular joint, 59, 61, **8.2**
Calculi
rhinoliths, 18, 25, **2.11**
submandibular duct stones, 65, **9.1**
of Wharton's duct, 66, **9.2**
Carcinoma
of dental alveolus, with mandibular invasion, 59, 64, **8.5**
of larynx, 85, 88–90, **13.4–13.6**
invading thyroid gland, 73, 77, **10.5**
of maxillary sinus, 19, 30, 32, **2.17, 2.19**
orbital invasion in, 41, 42, 44, **4.2, 4.4**
nasopharyngeal, 37–39, **3.1, 3.2**
intracranial extension of, 49, 50, **6.2**
of oral cavity, with mandibular invasion, 59, 63, **8.4**
of piriform sinus, metastasis of, 103, 105, **16.4**
of thyroid gland, 73, 76, **10.4**
lymph node metastasis of, 103, 106, **16.5**
of tongue base, 93, 95, **14.2**
of trachea, 85, 91, **13.8**
Carotid artery, internal, 1, 3, **1.1**
Carotid body tumor, 99, 100, **15.1**
Cerebrospinal fluid leak, in fracture of sphenoid sinus, 49, 51, **6.6**
Cochlea, 1, 3, **1.1**
Computed tomography
in acoustic neuroma, 2, 9, 10, **1.7–1.9**
in aryepiglottic fold arteriovenous malformation, 85, 90, **13.7**
in carotid body tumor, 99, 100, **15.1**
in cholesteatoma, 1, 5, **1.3**
in craniometaphyseal dysplasia, 53, 54, **7.1**
in facial nerve schwannoma, 2, 11, **1.10**
in frontoethmoid mucocele, 19, 26, **2.12**
in glomus jugulare tumor, 3, 14, **1.13**
in glomus vagale tumor, 99, 101, **15.2**
in goiter, with extension into mediastinum, 81, 82, **12.1**
in laryngeal carcinoma, 84, 88, 89, **13.4, 13.5**
invading thyroid gland, 73, 77, **10.5**
maxillary sinus
in carcinoma, 19, 30, 32, **2.17, 2.19**
in cysts, 17, 18, 21, 24, **2.6, 2.10**
in multiple myeloma, 109, 115, **17.3**
nasopharyngeal
in angiofibroma, 19, 29, **2.16**
in carcinoma, 37–39, **3.1, 3.2**
in olfactory esthesioneuroblastoma, 19, 31, **2.18**
in paranasal sinus papillomas, 18, 28, 29, **2.13–2.15**
in parotid gland disorders, 66, 69–72, **9.4–9.8**
in rhinoliths, 18, 25, **2.11**
in temporal bone osteomyelitis, 3, 16, **1.14**
in thyroid carcinoma, 73, 76, **10.4**
metastatic, 103, 106, **16.5**
in thyroid cyst extension to mediastinum, 81, 83, **12.2**
in tongue tumors, 93–95, **14.2, 14.3**
Craniometaphyseal dysplasia, 53, 54, **7.1**
Cyst
in maxillary sinus, 17, 18, 21, 24, **2.5–2.7, 2.10**
thyroglossal duct, 103, 104, **16.1**
thyroid, 73, 74, **10.1**
extension into mediastinum, 81, 83, **12.2**

Diverticulum, Zenker's, of hypopharynx, 93, 97, 98, **14.6, 14.7**

Dysplasia
    craniometaphyseal, 53, 54, **7.1**
    fibrous, skull, 45, 46, **5.1**

Ectasia, jugular venous, 99, 100, **15.3**
Embolization, transcatheter, in glomus jugulare tumor, 3, 14, **1.13**
Encephalocele
    ethmoid, 49, 51, **6.4**
    sphenoid, 49, 50, **6.3**
Epiglottitis, acute, 85, 86, **13.1**
Epitympanum, cholesteatoma of, 1, 4, **1.2**
Esthesioneuroblastoma, olfactory, 19, 31, **2.18**
    orbital extension of, 41, 43, **4.3**
Ethmoid sinus
    encephalocele, 49, 51, **6.4**
    osteoma with orbital extension, 41, **4.1**
    papilloma of, inverting, 18, 28, **2.14**

Facial nerve, 1, 3, **1.1**
    schwannoma of, 2, 11, **1.10**
Fistula, oroantral, 17, 20, **2.4**
Foramen magnum, 1, 3, **1.1**
Foramen ovale, 1, 3, **1.1**
    expansion by malignant schwannoma, 45, 46, **5.2**
Foramen rotundum, enlargement by neurofibroma, 45, 47, **5.3**
Foreign bodies, in hypopharynx, 93, 96, **14.5**
Fracture(s)
    facial, 53, 57, **7.4**
    Le Fort, 53, 57, **7.4**
    nasal, 53, 55, **7.2**
    orbital floor, 53, 56, **7.3**
    sphenoid sinus, cerebrospinal fluid leak in, 49, 51, **6.6**
    zygoma, 53, 56, **7.3**
Frontal sinus
    subfrontal meningioma in, 49, 51, **6.5**
    osteoma of, 17, 22, **2.8**
    sinusitis
        extradural abscess with, 49, **6.1**

        osteomyelitis with, 19, 35, 49, **2.20, 6.1**

Gastrointestinal tract
    hypopharynx and cervical esophagus, 93, 96–98, **14.5–14.7**
    oral cavity and pharynx, 93–96, **14.1–14.4**
    upper tract, 93–98, **14.1–14.7**
Geniculate ganglion, 1, 3, **1.1**
Glomus jugulare tumor, 2, 12, **1.11**
    intraarterial embolization of, 3, 14, **1.13**
Glomus vagale tumor, 99, 101, **15.2**
Goiter, mediastinal, 81, 82, **12.1**

Hemangioma, cavernous
    of parotid gland, 67, 72, **9.9**
    of tongue, 93, 95, **14.3**
Hyperparathyroidism, brown tumors in, 109, 110, **17.1**
Hypopharynx
    foreign body in, 93, 96, **14.5**
    Zenker's diverticulum, 93, 97, 98, **14.6, 14.7**

Incus, 1, 3, **1.1**

Jugular foramen, 1, 3, **1.1**
Jugular vein aneurysm, 99, 101, **15.3**

Larynx, 85–91
    arteriovenous malformation of aryepiglottic fold, 85, 90, **13.7**
    carcinoma of, 85, 88–90, **13.4–13.6**
        invading thyroid gland, 73, 77, **10.5**
    epiglottitis, acute, 85, 86, **13.1**
    internal laryngocele, 85, 86, **13.3**
    in multiple myeloma, 109, 115, **17.3**
    trauma of, 85, 86, **13.2**
Le Fort fractures of facial bones, 53, 57, **7.4**
Lingual thyroid gland, 93, 94, **14.1**
Lipoma
    of parotid gland, 66, 70, **9.6**
    of submandibular region, 103, 104, **16.2**

Lymph nodes, cervical
    in piriform sinus carcinoma metastasis, 103, 105, **16.4**
    in thyroid carcinoma metastasis, 103, 106, **16.5**

Magnetic resonance imaging
    in acoustic neuromas, bilateral, 3, 13, **1.12**
    in laryngeal carcinoma, 85, 90, **13.6**
    in maxillary sinus cyst, 17, 22, **2.7**
Mandible, 59–64, **8.1–8.5**
    invasion by alveolar carcinoma, 59, 64, **8.5**
    invasion by oral cavity carcinoma, 59, 63, **8.4**
    osteosarcoma of, 59, 62, **8.3**
    osteomyelitis of, 59, 62, **8.1**
Mastoid bone, in cholesteatoma, 1, 4, 6, **1.2, 1.4**
Maxillary sinus
    air–fluid level in, 17, 21, **2.5**
    carcinoma of, 19, 30, 32, **2.17, 2.19**
        intracranial extension of, 45, 48–50, **5.5, 6.2**
        orbital invasion of, 41, 42, 44, **4.2, 4.4**
    cysts in, 17, 18, 21, 22, **2.5–2.7**
        dentigerous, 18, 24, **2.10**
        retention, 17, 18, 21, 22, **2.5–2.7**
    papilloma of, inverting, 18, 28, **2.13**
    purulent sinusitis
        acute, 17, 19, **2.2**
        chronic, 17, 18, 23, **2.9**
Maxillofacial skeleton, 53–57, **7.1–7.4**
    craniometaphyseal dysplasia, 53, 54, **7.1**
    trauma of, 53, 55–57, **7.2–7.4**
Mediastinum
    superior, 81–83, **12.1, 12.2**
        goiter extension into, 81, 82, **12.1**
        thyroid cyst extension into, 81, 83, **12.2**
Meningioma, subfrontal, in orbit and

frontal sinuses, 49, 51, **6.5**
Mucocele, frontoethmoid, 19, 26,
2.12
Mucoepidermoid tumor, malignant,
of parotid gland, 66, 72, **9.8**
Multiple myeloma, larynx in, 109,
115, **17.3**

Nasal bones, fracture of, 53, 55, **7.2**
Nasopharynx
carcinoma of, 37–39, **3.1, 3.2**
intracranial extension of, 49,
50, **6.1**
tumors of, 19, 29, 37–39, **2.16,
3.1, 3.2**
Neurofibroma, foramen rotundum
enlargement in, 45, 47, **5.3**
Neuroma, acoustic, 2, 9, 10,
1.7–1.9
bilateral, 3, 13, **1.12**

Olfactory esthesioneuroblastoma,
19, 31, **2.18**
orbital extension of, 41, 43, **4.3**
Oral cavity, 93–95, **14.1–14.3**
carcinoma of, with mandibular
invasion, 59, 63, **8.4**
Orbit
fractures of floor, 53, 56, **7.3**
invasion by diseases, 41–44,
4.1–4.4
in ethmoid osteoma, 41, **4.1**
in maxillary sinus carcinoma,
41, 42, 44, **4.2, 4.4**
in olfactory esthesioneuroblastoma, 41, 43, **4.3**
subfrontal meningioma in, 49,
51, **6.5**
Osteoma
ethmoid, with orbital invasion,
41, **4.1**
frontal sinus, 17, 22, **2.8**
Osteomyelitis
frontal sinusitis with, 19, 35, 49,
2.20, 6.1
of mandible, 59, 60, **8.1**
of temporal bone, 3, 16, **1.14**
Osteosarcoma, of mandible, 59, 62,
8.3
Otorhinologic disorders, intracranial
extension of, 49–51, **6.1–6.6**

Paget's disease of bone, cranial
changes in, 109, 113, **17.2**
Papilloma, inverting
of ethmoid sinus, 18, 28, **2.14**
of maxillary sinus, 18, 28, **2.13**
of sphenoid sinus and nasal cavity, 18, 29, **2.15**
Paranasal sinuses, 17–23, **2.1–2.9**
See also Sinuses, paranasal
Parathyroid glands, 79, 80, **11.1, 11.2**
adenoma of, 79, 80, **11.1**
thyroid adenoma with, 79, 80,
11.2
Parotid gland
abscess of, 66, 69, **9.4**
benign mixed tumor of, 66, 71,
9.7
cavernous hemangioma of, 67,
72, **9.9**
fatty infiltration of, 66, 69, **9.5**
lipoma of, 66, 70, **9.6**
malignant mucoepidermoid
tumor of, 66, 72, **9.8**
Warthin's tumor of, 65, 68, **9.3**
Petrosal nerve, 1, 2, **1.1**
Pharynx, 93–96, **14.1–14.4.** *See
also* Hypopharynx; Nasopharynx
retropharyngeal abscess, 93, 96,
14.4
Piriform sinus carcinoma, metastasis
of, 103, 105, **16.4**
Pott's puffy tumor, frontal sinusitis
with, 49, **6.1**
Pseudogout of temporomandibular
joint, 59, 61, **8.2**

Retropharyngeal abscess, 93, 96,
14.4
Rhinoliths, 18, 25, **2.11**
Rhinorrhea, cerebrospinal fluid, in
fracture of sphenoid sinus, 49, 51,
6.6

Salivary glands, 65–72, **9.1–9.9**
multiple submandibular duct
stones, 65, **9.1**
sialectasis, submandibular, 65,
66, **9.2**
Schuller projection, temporal bone,
1, 3, **1.1**

Schwannoma
of facial nerve, 2, 11, **1.10**
malignant
foramen ovale expansion in,
45, 46, **5.2**
of trigeminal nerve, 45, 48, **5.4**
of spinal accessory nerve, 103,
104, **16.3**
Scintigraphy
of brown tumors in hyper-
parathyroidism, 109, 110, **17.1**
of fibrous dysplasia of skull, 45,
46, **5.1**
of frontal sinusitis with
osteomyelitis, 19, 35, **2.20**
of goiter extension into superior
mediastinum, 81, 82, **12.1**
of lingual thyroid gland, 93, 94,
14.1
of mandibular osteosarcoma, 59,
62, **8.3**
of mandibular osteomyelitis, 59,
60, **8.1**
of maxillary sinus carcinoma, 19,
32, **2.19**
of multiple myeloma, 109, 115,
17.3
of oral cavity carcinoma with
mandibular invasion, 59, 63,
8.4
of Paget's disease, 109, 113,
17.2
of parotid gland cavernous
hemangioma, 67, 72, **9.9**
of piriform sinus carcinoma
metastasis, 103, 105, **16.4**
of temporal bone osteomyelitis,
3, 16, **1.14**
of thyroid adenoma, 73–75,
10.2, 10.3
of thyroid carcinoma, 73, 76,
10.4
of Warthin's tumor of parotid
gland, 65, 68, **9.3**
Scutum, 1, 3, **1.1**
Semicircular canals, 1, 3, **1.1**
Sialectasis, submandibular, 66, 67,
9.2
Sinuses, paranasal, 17–23, **2.1–2.9**
in angiofibroma of nasopharynx,
19, 29, **2.16**

frontoethmoid mucocele, 19, 26,
2.12
in olfactory esthesioneuroblastoma, 19, 31, **2.18**
oroantral fistula, 17, 20, **2.4**
papillomas of, inverting, 18, 28,
29, **2.13–2.15**
radiologic signs of disease in, 17,
2.1
rhinoliths, 18, 25, **2.11**
sphenoiditis, acute purulent, 17,
19, **2.3**. *See also* Sphenoid
sinus
Skull
base of
evaluation of, 45–48, **5.1–5.5**
in fibrous dysplasia, 45, 46,
5.1
in foramen ovale expansion
by malignant schwannoma,
45, 46, **5.2**
in foramen rotundum enlargement by neurofibroma, 45,
47, **5.3**
in maxillary sinus carcinoma
with intracranial extension,
45, 48, **5.5**
in trigeminal schwannoma,
malignant, 45, 48, **5.4**
craniometaphyseal dysplasia, 53,
54, **7.1**
Paget's disease of, 109, 113,
17.2
Soft-tissue lesions of neck, 103–107,
16.1–16.5
Sonography
in maxillary sinusitis, 17, 18, 23,
2.9
of parathyroid adenoma, 79, 80,
11.1, 11.2
of thyroid adenoma, 73, 75,
10.2
of thyroid carcinoma metastasis,
103, 106, **16.5**
of thyroid cyst, 73, 74, **10.1**
Sphenoid sinus
encephalocele, 49, 50, **6.3**
fracture of, cerebrospinal fluid
leak in, 49, 51, **6.6**
papilloma of, inverting, 18, 29,
2.15

Sphenoiditis, acute purulent, 17, 29,
2.3
Stapes, 1, 3, **1.1**
Submandibular duct stones, 65, **9.1**
Submandibular gland
lipoma in region of, 103, 104,
16.2
sialectasis, 66, 67, **9.2**
Systemic disorders, 109–115,
17.1–17.3

Temporal bone, 1–16, **1.1–1.14**
in acoustic neuroma, 2, 9, 10,
13, **1.7–1.9, 1.12**
in bony atresia of auditory canal,
2, 8, **1.6**
in cholesteatoma, 1, 4–6, **1.2–1.4**
in fracture through external auditory canal, 1, 7, **1.5**
in glomus jugulare tumor, 2, 3,
12, 14, **1.11, 1.13**
in osteomyelitis, 3, 16, **1.14**
in schwannoma of facial nerve,
2, 11, **1.10**
Temporomandibular joint, pseudogout of, 59, 61, **8.2**
Thyroglossal duct cyst, 103, 104,
16.1,
Thyroid gland, 73–77, **10.1–10.5**
adenoma of, 73–75, 79, 80,
10.2, 10.3, 11.2
parathyroid adenoma with,
79, 80, **11.2**
carcinoma of, 73, 76, **10.4**
lymph node metastasis of,
103, 106, **16.5**
cyst of, 73, 74, **10.1**
extension into superior mediastinum, 81, 83, **12.2**
goiter extension into mediastinum, 81, 82, **12.1**
invasion by carcinoma of larynx,
73, 77, **10.5**
lingual, 93, 94, **14.1**
Tomograms
complex-motion
in cholesteatoma, 1, 2, 5–9,
1.3–1.7
in foramen rotundum enlargement by neurofibroma, 45,
47, **5.3**

in glomus jugulare tumor, 2,
12, **1.11**
in maxillary sinus carcinoma,
19, 32, **2.19**
in maxillary sinus cyst,
dentigerous, 18, 24, **2.10**
in temporomandibular pseudogout, 59, 61, **8.2**
panoramic
in mandibular osteomyelitis,
59, 60, **8.1**
in maxillary sinus carcinoma,
19, 32, **2.19**
in oral cavity carcinoma with
mandibular invasion, 59, 63,
8.4
Tongue
carcinoma of base, 93, 95,
14.2
cavernous hemangioma of, 93,
95, **14.3**
lingual thyroid gland, 93, 94,
14.1
Trachea
carcinoma of, 85, 91, **13.8**
cervical, 85
Trauma. *See also* Fracture(s)
laryngeal, 85, 86, **13.2**
maxillofacial, 53, 55–57, **7.2–
7.4**
Tumors. *See also specific tumor
types*
carotid body, 99, 100, **15.1**
glomus vagale, 99, 101, **15.2**
nasopharyngeal, 19, 29, 37–39,
2.16, 3.1, 3.2

Vasculature. *See also specific vessels*
head and neck lesions, 99–101,
15.1–15.3
Vestibule of ear, 1, 3, **1.1**

Warthin's tumor of parotid gland,
65, 68, **9.3**
Wharton's duct, stenosis and calculus of, 66, 67, **9.2**

Zenker's diverticulum of hypopharynx, 93, 97, 98, **14.6, 14.7**
Zygoma, fracture of, 53, 56, **7.3**